A CANTERBURY TALE

A

CANTERBURY TALE

The Autobiography of
Dr Francis Bennett

Oxford University Press
Wellington

Oxford University Press
OXFORD LONDON GLASGOW
NEW YORK TORONTO MELBOURNE WELLINGTON
KUALA LUMPUR SINGAPORE HONG KONG TOKYO
NAIROBI DAR ES SALAAM CAPE TOWN
DELHI BOMBAY CALCUTTA MADRAS KARACHI

ISBN 0 19 558065 6

Photoset in Bembo and printed by
Whitcoulls Ltd, Christchurch
Published by Oxford University Press,
222-236 Willis Street,
Wellington, New Zealand

'With us ther was a Doctour of Phisik'
Chaucer, *The Canterbury Tales*

CONTENTS

ILLUSTRATIONS

1

Not In Entire Forgetfulness

The man was bent low as he picked his way across the stone-littered paddock, carrying the gun at the slope. The boy watched from the verandah, tense, gripping the post with sweating hands and white knuckles. Ahead of the man was a prism of stones fifteen yards long and five feet high. In its shadow he suddenly stood erect and raised the gun. From the ambush of the rotting sheep the hawk heaved itself lazily into the air, flapping towards safety on the other side of the pines. The gun, now a thin black rod slowly swung round, jerked and was lowered. The wings of the bird crumpled; it lost height and then with fearsome acceleration pitched to the ground. The hens, terrified and screeching, raced for the shelter of the trees. On the verandah the boy jumped and yelled as excitement had to translate itself into noise.

It was one of the expressions of my father's might that he could wave a black wand at a bird and it would fall dead. I had no idea that some lead particles intervened. But somehow he seemed to confirm that together we had despatched the chicken-stealing hawk. Later, in my fourth year, I was allowed to put the gun away behind the door. It was enormously heavy and one barrel was warm and one cold. Its smell was neither pleasant nor unpleasant, just exciting.

The earliest memories were of violence. Yet I always triumphed over the violence and by the age of four my egotism and self-confidence were such that no malign influence could reach me. I filled my pensive moments with magnificent deeds lacking all detail except that they were fulsomely praised by my parents. I strutted about the kitchen floor, shoving chairs aside, lurched down the two steps at the back door, descended (backwards) from the high front verandah, made the dog get out of my way. I must have been an intolerable little twerp. Like Alexander Selkirk I was monarch of all I surveyed. But while he surveyed an island I surveyed a three-roomed house and its weedy environs. My world however was more populous. Against his one man I had two parents and at a later date the resented insidious arrival of a brother.

His advent made the small house even smaller. But there was another house across the creek, a sort of shepherd's hut. There came a morning when some strange men came to breakfast and I was continually told to keep out of the way. Then they disappeared. My mother was shut in her room and I was alone in the world. An instinct told me that what I sought was on the other side of the creek, up the cliff and over the ridge. So there I went crawling under the lowest wire, skirting the yard, crossing the creek on the fallen log (strictly forbidden), meandering through bog and flax bushes and dragging on tussocks while clambering up the cliff. Finally, breathless, I sprawled over the edge and looked around.

There, momentarily I stayed, rooted with terror. The monster was bearing down on me from a distance which I now know to be about a chain. It was spouting smoke and flames, clanking and lumbering with malign intent. Its front was an enormous circular plate, obviously a maw, ready to open when I was within reach. It had already captured the shepherd's hut and some men were trying to prevent the removal by placing long round logs in front. My father shouted at me. I ran downhill and away from the cliff. I turned round. It had changed direction and was following me. Back to the cliff edge and as I slipped over I saw it swerve again in my direction. On the flat I twisted in and out among the flax, shook off the pursuit and finally reached home. Late in the afternoon, still shaking, I watched from afar the traction engine straining on the ropes, the men, hammering and shouting, and finally the juxtaposition of the two buildings. An achievement certainly. Even a four-year-old could sense that, but I had paid a price. Fear had now been added to the emotional tangle.

But this was my home and I remember very little about it. The verandah was too high for me to mount and my only access was up the steps at the back door and through the house. The kitchen table was covered with torn American oil-cloth. Somewhere a wall was lined with newspapers. My bedroom (shared alas) had yellow and brown wallpaper, with endless repetitions of the rural fantasy of a wagon and two cows under a willow tree. It was scrim based and it bellied with every wind. The house became known in the district as 'Bennett's folly'. This seemed to please my father. Apparently the criticism of neighbours was preferable to their indifference.

In the house was my mother but she was of little account. Most of the time she was in bed or occasionally in a chair on castors. We soon learned her little ways: that she could not follow up her orders and that if we were out of sight or out of sound we were safe; that at times she would be found crying ('Because of the pain,' explained my father, using a word not yet in our vocabulary); that if we came too near she might ask us to kiss her which we did reluctantly bending over precariously so as not to touch her painful arms. We knew she was our mother, whatever that meant. Like Kipling's character we learned about women from her. We learned that all women were sedentary, tearful, demanding and generally ineffective. They may have had other qualities because, paradoxically, we sought her favour and warmed to her praise.

My father of course was God; not the God who rode invisibly on one's shoulder and who used a very black pencil to note down all misdemeanours, but an all-powerful God of action, who could break in a young horse, kill a sheep, stride fearlessly through the cow yard, shoot a hawk, fell a tree, fold my mother in his arms and carry her off to bed. These were the true tests of manhood.

No one passed the house for it was at the end of a side road. No other houses were in sight. Sometimes my father, who of course had absolute freedom of the world, would drive off in the trap and become part of the bluish haze over the distant trees. 'He'll be back before dark,' my mother would assure me. 'We live in the backblocks, you know.' This I came to realize meant remoteness from other centres of world population such as Geraldine, Timaru, Christchurch and London. Even Woodbury was practically inaccessible being over two miles away.

At the age of three or maybe four I was involved in a clamorous non-event. It concerned the fire. The flames engulfed the building, swirling to reveal the scarlet, the mauve and the grey. There was the snap and sparkle against the steady roar from the doomed structure. At times the smoke would fling a screen across and then the screen would be a shower of sparks. There were no fire brigades, no spectators other than me, no fear, no identification of the burning building.

So much for the fire and now for the mystery. For the fire was a dream and it was a dream based on nothing. My parents were confident I had seen no great fire, no burning building, no straw stack, no gorse fire, no tussock burning. Nothing but the resinous pine slabs reddening at the edges in the old wood stove. I have seen plenty of fires since, from the one in the gorse fence near the school started through my misjudging the potential of a match, to the inferno of an exploding ammunition dump in Guadalcanal. But none of them were more authentic or more vivid than the fire of the dream, nor as well remembered to the present day. My parents were impressed with my confident descriptions. 'He must have the second sight,' commented a visitor, determined not to waste a good phrase. But my parents rejected this. There was nothing about second sight in the New Testament. So the mystery remained and is a mystery still.

Another event with traumatic overtones was the arrival of my brother – not the one next to me but the one after. Though I, more or less, slept through it, yet the details still persist. I was then, on the authority of the Registrar-General aged three years six weeks and four days. It had been a strange day. There were two foreign women in the house and they made it plain they were not there to please me. Even my father seemed to defer to them. In the small hours of the morning when my sleep was so deep as to be almost irremediable, one of these women shook me and kept on shaking saying, 'Come on, come on, your mother wants you to see your little baby brother.' Waking was an agony. My little baby brother was an unpardonable intrusion. She dragged me down the short passage into the last room on the right. In the corner facing the door my mother was sitting up incongruously alert and smiling. I was taken to the other corner and lifted up to peer into a cot. In the depths of the clothing something stirred. I was lifted up to kiss my mother. I remembered my unqualified resentment at this trespass on my nocturnal rights but I do not remember going back to bed. I suppose by then I was sleep walking. A fig for young brothers. If it was a question of his existence or my repose I at least had the rights of a senior.

Somewhere, as the years rolled on from four through five the other three members of the household were reappraised. My mother was perhaps not quite as ineffective as I had once thought. She would tease us, laugh with us, read us stories. We were sorry she had the painful joints, but it was dutiful sorrow, like sorrow at a lost ball or a wet day. In her helplessness we had to be her hands and feet and whenever we came within earshot she had a mission ready. Though we could have defied her with impunity we rarely did. We preferred her favour which meant of course the additional favour of father.

My brother was still a pest but a pest with a personality. Life coloured up when he was around. One day he tottered into the kitchen screaming, his face covered with blood. It was my first encounter with this substance, my first lesson in haematology. The family cat had at last taken a stand. I went out, a veritable St George, to do battle to the death with the cat. I passed my father going in. Shortly afterwards, carrying the gun, he found me in the yard. 'Go inside boy and stay there.' Ten minutes later he came back. 'Oh, did you have to?' said my mother in distress. 'The boy could have lost his eyes,' he said tersely. He handed me the gun to put away. As usual one barrel was warm.

I remember the calamitous incident of the bath. My brother had gone outside after a week's remand, and had found an irresistible attraction in a pool of mud and slush. He arrived back whimpering as well he might for he was a black, dripping, repulsive figure. My mother, appalled, immediately prescribed a bath and this of necessity involved me. I dragged in the tin bath, added, as she directed, the hot and cold. The hot water came from the tin kettle on the stove for the old black one was too heavy. The cold water came from the tap in the tank at the back door. How the temperature was regulated I do not know. Then I had to undress the object. He resisted and began to bawl. I was angry and resentful, furious with him and furious with my mother. But I could not get him into the bath. She seemed to have more regard for him than for me. I began to cry at the gross humiliation and injustice of it all. Then to my astonishment my mother let her head fall forward and began to sob. So there we were, all crying: the filthy midget, the haughty brother, the frustrated mother. Then the door opened. My father stood there, tall, black-bearded, dominant. What a man! Before my mother could explain he was in action. While my brother was squirming at being tickled he was plonked in the bath. My mother was swept off to the bedroom. I was soon racing happily on a variety of missions. Wood was jammed in the stove, food was processed into pots and pans, and a roast was discovered in the oven. My mother came back, now smiling. My brother, miraculously clean and dry, was turned loose. The dirty clothes, the bath, the towel all disappeared. Soon we were all up at the table deep in good rich food, everyone a-simmer with cordiality.

My father was certainly all things to all men – confident and competent as in the incident just described, lowly and reverent in the grace before meals, daring and intrepid before the rearing horse, the threatening bull, the crash and splash of the dray as it plunged down and up again across the bed of the creek. In a quite different mood he put us to bed, bantering and boisterous, and insisting on hilarious impossibilities of conduct.

One night this procedure revealed him in an astonishing new potential. My brother and I slept together in a square bed with wooden slats covered by a chaff mattress. Our bed-chamber technique was to stand in the middle of the mattress, disrobe and toss the garments on the floor. On this night our father's good humour had evoked in us a mischievous response. I, half undressed, said 'Let's scream.' Immediately my brother began to scream. I joined in. It was a glorious noise, scream after scream after scream. My parents' bedroom was next door. I expected a gruff command to stop, but there was silence only, silence, that is, for a short time. We went on screaming. Suddenly the door was flung open with a violence that nearly cost it the hinges. My father burst into the room. His hair was tousled, he was clad in a singlet and long woollen underpants. He crouched in true simian fashion. In his raised right hand was a heavy lump of wood. We were immediately astonished and silent. I forget how it all ended, which meant that there was nothing remarkable in the adjustment. But we never screamed again.

It is only in retrospect that the stature of my father can be fully seen. Unaided he controlled a poor farm: crops, sheep, cows, pigs and poultry. Unaided he nursed my mother and ran the house. Who did the cooking, the cleaning, the washing? Often I would be sent by my mother to hang the white towel over the gate of the yard. Then he would tie the team up and come striding home to her aid. She did all the sewing for she was an expert needlewoman. She also did most of the washing up with all the dishes in an enamel basin, laboriously washing and drying them one by one.

These dull days were occasionally transformed by the arrival after breakfast and departure before tea of either my father's mother who lived at Fairfield a few miles over the hills, or his elder sister, my Aunt Katie, whose husband farmed at Te Moana further on still. I remember them as being blackclad, soft-spoken, kindly to small boys but exacting certain standards of conduct: not to step on wet floors, nor to touch the clothes-prop supporting the wet washing, not to hang around the kitchen during the baking, and to keep a steady supply of cones for the fire. If a blameless day resulted we were rewarded with two currant buns, hot from the oven.

It was hard to get away from my brother. I remember spending most of an afternoon on and off the bars of a gate confident that my father's prophecy would be fulfilled. And it was. A mile away the main road was hidden by the gorse fence but at last through the gaps could be seen a white object which kept flicking in and out of sight. We raced into my mother. 'We saw it, we saw it, we saw it.' Our jubilation was shrilled up with the excitement of seeing our first car. We challenged her as to whether she had seen one. She was evasive and we concluded she had not. Our triumph deepened.

Of necessity we had to make our own amusements. My brother had a beloved wooden doll called Judy which he treated scandalously so that it was charred in the fire, thrown in the creek, buried in the mud and run over by the dray. Each calamity signified a contemptuous rejection by the owner, to be followed, sometimes months later, by an ecstatic reunion even though Judy eventually had the form and features of a piece of kindling. We exploited to the full the resources of the wheelbarrow. When upside down the wheel would spin freely and even furiously when the flax rope wound round the axle was pulled. It bore a happy resemblance to the flywheel of a threshing machine and a threshing machine it became. An inclined board was erected above the wheel and up the board, with appropriate sounds we pushed wisps of straw. Embellishments were excitedly added. The most successful was the nail driven through the board which when lowered onto the rotating wheel shrieked intolerably though to us it was the sweet call of the engine's whistle to morning tea. My father was very amused and gave us a list of farmers needing our services. So we threshed our way round Woodbury and presumably were in charge of a very contented gang, for most of their working hours were spent in answering the summons for morning tea.

For a period (I being then about five), my father rode in to the Woodbury store every Saturday evening nominally to collect the mail, which normally consisted of household pamphlets revealing specific cures for all disease. Actually it was his escape session from the stress of the week. Saturday night was the farmers' night at the store and all the news of the week, the triumphs, and the calamities were laid out and shared. (My father was much amused over the boast of an illiterate neighbour that his lambing season had returned him one hundred and twenty per cent among the singles.) In the store was a rifle-range extending from the door to the dimly lit targets on the row of full sacks at the far end. Here every Saturday evening there was for an hour or so the plop-plop-plop of .22 ammunition willingly sold by the indulgent store-keeper. But vastly more important to us was that each Saturday he brought home a new issue of *Comic Cuts*. This was read to us by my mother on the Sunday evening. It was our highlight of the week and they must have recognized this by allowing such frivolity on a Sunday. The hero of the periodical was Tiger Tim (animal, not human, though it was a close shave). Each week he would become involved in extraordinary escapades from which he always emerged triumphantly to our astonishment and delight. One Sunday evening when my brother and I confronted my mother across the kitchen table she announced that her red inflamed eyes made it impossible for her to conduct the session. So I offered to read and in due course did. Tiger Tim was perhaps not as slick as usual but he got there. Thereafter my mother or I did the reading. Not long after, my brother was admitted to the reading partnership. School for me was still nearly three years away. I have no memory of ever learning to read. Nor has my brother.

Writing was equally mysterious, for at the age of six I began to write a novel. It was not the writing but the obsession to write that was the puzzling feature. I had never read a novel and I had no acquaintance with any literature beyond the Bible, *Comic Cuts*, pamphlets on Mother Seagull's Syrup, Doan's backache kidney pills, Dr Williams' pink pills, and a variety of tracts where a snappy introduction would be the lure to some moral issue. My title was 'The Adventures of a Half Sovereign' (in an amended version it became a full sovereign). It had a well constructed plot. It was told by the coin itself in the first person. In the opening chapter the excitement mounted as the sovereign heard the miner's pick getting nearer and nearer, then fading along false trails, surging with hope again as the sounds grew louder. (I had no reason to believe that gold was found in other than minted form.) But the miner at last unearthed the coin and the next day spent it (possibly to buy a farm or a team, for I had no idea of the value of money). Thereafter the plot was to hinge on an endless series of transactions leaving an endless series of gratified purchasers. One afternoon a neighbour's trap brought two women to visit my mother. They sat on the verandah and one of the visitors made tea. They held no interest for me and I went off to my novel. I was now half way through the second exercise book. (The first had been mislaid somewhere.) After the tea there was loud laughter and I crept nearer. To my horror my mother was reading my novel aloud. My shame and humiliation were almost unbearable. Late that afternoon I retrieved it and shoved both volumes into the stove. It was an appropriate end for a bad book and a fine example for all second-rate novelists.

Even stranger was an essay into verse. I announced the result to my mother.

> I climbed a tree
> And caught a bee.

'Very good,' she said patting me on the head. 'Now go and make up some more.'

I made up some more and offered it to her:

> I climbed a tree
> And caught a bee
> And saw the sea.

'Yes,' said my mother, 'but I liked the first one better.'

So, actually, did I. The revised version had expanded the scope but forfeited the continuity of the narrative. So the third line was scrapped. It was again a valuable lesson which some more experienced versifiers might well follow.

This incident invites two comments. Firstly, why was a verse form selected? Admittedly there was no Miltonic ring about the lines but they did follow the hearty old John Bull tradition of rhythm and rhyme. There were no books of poetry in the house. Tiger Tim conversed only in extravagant prose. Presumably the idea must have come from Moody and Sankey's hymns ('Pull for the shore, sailor' and 'Where is my wandering boy tonight?'). The second comment concerns my vivid recollection of my mother. She was standing, clutching the kitchen table with both hands. She released the right hand to pat me on the head. It was the only time I can remember her standing.

Such memories survive because they are based on a traumatic foundation. A gun, a traction engine, a cat, a fire, a bath, a night alarm, a public humiliation. The danger loomed, the alarm bells rang, there was survival and the lessons from the survival were carefully stored away, and easily resurrected at a new crisis. Man can never lack interest in disaster. Bad news is always real news.

I was once taken by my father to the 1905 Exhibition in Hagley Park. Two vivid memories of that day remain – one based on fear, and one on wonder. The first one was the water chute where all day long the intrepid ones were hurled twenty thousand leagues under the sea and yet returned smiling, dry and unscathed.

But the more dramatic discovery that day was West's Pictures, most appropriately called 'The Flicks'. They had been seen at Dunedin a few months before as part of a concert programme. The first motion picture had been in Paris ten years earlier. In New Zealand they had been presented occasionally in vaudeville. But West's Pictures at the Exhibition represented the first complete cinema performance. The films were all shorts which guaranteed many houses in a day.

I had never heard of pictures that could move. I was looking at pure magic and any criticism would have been vulgar. It was a cogwheel splutter of stills but I saw it as a smooth sequence of animation. Even stills were extraordinary enough and a popular amusement at the time was a magic lantern show. Much earlier I had attended a public lecture by the eccentric Professor Bickerton. My aunt took me but probably under instructions from my grandfather. The lecturer had his lantern on a table halfway down the aisle and I sat nearly behind it with a very poor view of the screen. I have no memory of the lecturer except that he carried a long pointer, moved up and down between lantern and screen and talked incessantly. But I remembered the fascination of the projected pictures of stars, the night sky faithfully reproduced in a dark hall.

The plot of that first film has never left me. It began with the baker leaving a loaf of bread at the castle gates and I gave no thought to the incongruity of quantity or place. Then a sinister-looking individual with a cap pulled down and a collar turned up stole the loaf. The butler after much handwringing as if he were a puppet with rusty joints put up a notice: 'Wanted – a watch dog'. The next day he was mobbed at the gate by hundreds of dogs all equipped with owners intent on transferring custody. He fled with dogs and men in pursuit. The long black canine line thinned to a thread on the distant hills. Did they catch him? I never knew. It was so wonderful in itself that it hardly mattered.

The mystery of human memory remains unsolved while the search for data goes on. These anecdotal trivia offer little to the search but throw some light on the life we led at Woodbury and it was a good life. We were isolated and our only contacts were with the indulgent Aunt Katie and Granny Bennett, the swaggering nonchalance (reciprocated) of the farmers for whom we did our imaginary threshing, the aggressiveness of Tiger Tim and the bland subservience of Judy. But we had a strong bond with our parents. We were healthy and busy, unaware of our deprivation or of the inevitable danger of introversion. Our environment declared our destiny. We were to be sturdy little farmers, meriting no more and deserving no less.

2

Convergence on Canterbury

Sometimes in the early days an atlas would be produced. 'This is where I used to live,' my mother would say, the long thin stick in her frozen fingers hovering over a map of London. Maps taught us nothing. They are subtle and ingenious and a four-year-old boy who claims to understand them is either a genius or a liar.

The only proved localities were Woodbury and Fairfield, for we had been there and had verified their existence. But the other places of which we heard – Orari, Pleasant Valley, Timaru, Geraldine, Christchurch and of course London – were imaginative ideas only, lacking material substance, like x and y or the Golden City of St Mary.

Fairfield was the name of my grandfather's farm a few miles over the hills. Two buildings confronted one another. One was a traditional farmhouse, the other a long low bunk-room for my uncles. These were surrounded by various outbuildings and animal enclosures – a conglomeration as formless as the pattern of a city when the cyclone has passed. In and out my grandfather and his sons strode purposefully followed by arrogant sheep dogs maintaining the affectation of great exertion by a lolling tongue and a panting breath. They seemed to have a limited emotional range – aggression to strangers, tolerance to children and a contempt for sheep.

Of the personalities which brought this confusion to life the most prominent was the tall, unsmiling, blackbearded man who came and went, gave authoritative orders and who looked at me as if he could never fathom the reason for my existence. Then there was his partner, the gracious lady with the buoyant lilt to her voice who could take a distressed small boy, let him hide his misery in her lap and convince him that he was safe with her till his mother or father returned. My uncles were young men with brusque manners and long strides like their father but with clean-shaven faces. They were more concerned with their horses and dogs than with me but they nodded and occasionally winked. A wink is a reassuring thing. It means you are not overlooked despite the handicap of one eye. I was to learn later that my father was the oldest of these brothers.

I also had two shadowy aunts one at each end of the family. At times of family crisis (my mother, for instance, being at Rotorua) I would reside temporarily at Fairfield. It was an exciting place with men and animals, implements, activity and noise. At the side of the house was the yard sloping steeply to a duckpond and up the other side was a gorse and blackberry slope spattered with gooseberry bushes.

My grandfather had a strong taste for adventure, especially if he had a credulous audience. Hear him tell it – born in Chester, England in 1840. At the age of fourteen a confrontation with his schoolmaster resulted in the latter being knocked unconscious by an ebony ruler. The next day he left his home (down the drain pipe) and his country (as cabin-boy), both permanently. Then for some years as an able seaman, in sail, he roamed the world, the monotony being relieved by friendships and fights, cyclones and shipwrecks, mutinies and desertion. At Sydney he knocked the first mate overboard. He followed, but from the other side. When well north of Sydney he was asked for the identity papers he did not have. The inference was that he was either a runaway sailor or an escaped convict. He chose the latter and for a time worked in a convict gang. But the truth could not be hidden; locked in a cabin in another ship he eventually reached Lyttelton, where he saw his old ship with the mate striding the deck. That night, with another man, he escaped and landed in New Zealand by crawling up through the marine mud like his prehistoric ancestors. The date was 1858 and this qualified me, so I have been informed, for membership of the Early Settlers' Association – but I doubt if the date would be strong enough if the circumstances were known. Thereafter the pace quickens: a race for the security of Otago, the convicts splashing across the Waitaki just ahead of the pursuit. Gabriel's Gully, money made and money lost, return to Canterbury, police curiosity and a trudge to the safety of the West Coast. At the Bealey Hotel was Burgess of the Burgess-Kelly Gang. He and my grandfather each sought the favour of a certain young lady, a guest at the hotel. The matter was settled by the approved method of the times, with bare fists. It finished with Burgess being knocked unconscious. The next day he vanished. The young lady became my grandmother. Then came West Coast adventures. Burgess determined to add Bill Bennett to his list of murders, might have succeeded if the hangman had not intervened at Nelson. Then my grandfather returned to Canterbury, married, settled at Arowhenua (Temuka) near Geraldine and thereafter lived at peace with all men provided they approached him with caution. A pretty tale deserving to be retold with awe. As a matter of high adventure all it lacked was proof. No one could vouch for it except my grandmother who came on the stage in the last act. Despite her zeal for the truth she never contradicted it. My father believed it and so did his siblings. But the story has been marred and pitted by history. In the *Cyclopaedia of Canterbury* (where is an awkward photo of him and some of his family) he is reputed to have arrived in New Zealand in the *North Star*. (There is no record of this ship in Lyttelton that year, though a wrong name might have been selected to thwart police curiosity.)

But no historical twisting can give any semblance of truth to the Burgess story. Burgess arrived in Otago in January 1862 having been released three months before from an Australian prison. My grandfather on 6 December 1861 married Mary Foley (a minor) at St Mary's Church, Timaru. The official evidence for this cannot be disputed. The bridegroom was a bushman. The witnesses were William Warne and Margaret Patterson. The minister was Rev. George Foster, the first vicar of the church which had been consecrated seven months before.

So the story falls if Burgess is in it. But if in the interests of dramatic effect the name of Burgess was substituted for a lesser antagonist there could be truth in the account and also in the rest of the narrative. Certainly my grandfather was never meant for a quiet life. When he was dying in Christchurch in 1923, being then eighty-three, he stormed deliriously every night, attempting impossible missions and fighting old fights. I, one of a series of voluntary night attendants, often sat up with him. One night I noticed a long and deep scar in his left flank. In the morning when he was rational I asked him about it.

'Oh, that? A scratch with a knife. Bit of a mutiny at sea. And none of your business, young fellow.'

This was hardly death-bed cordiality but at least it was an improvement. In my earliest sojourns at Fairfield he ignored me except occasionally at meal times when he would startle me with 'Eat up boy. Eat up and give the ship a good name'. Then there came an occasion, yet to be told, where he and I were involved in a matter of a firearm and after that we ceased to communicate.

Marriage put an end to his roving and he settled in Pleasant Valley near Geraldine. From there he operated a bullock team carting wool by contract out of the Mackenzie country. He also (according to the official history of South Canterbury) ran a boarding house for saw-millers. It is much more likely that his wife controlled it leaving him on his periodic returns to deal with the complaints and the bad debts.

Most of the land within the vicinity was held under pastoral lease by members of the Tripp and Elsworthy families. But from about 1860 onwards a steady selling programme was followed.

One Crown grant in Pleasant Valley of nearly fifty acres (Rural Section 3607) was made on 9 May 1864 to William Campion. This was in the week that my father was born. Twelve years later my grandfather bought half of it from Campion and within a year the other half from William Grace. And he at the age of thirty-six with a wife and seven children established himself as a freehold farmer – a sailor truly home from the sea.

Surely a minor event, magnified in this record – fifty acres, not only in the backblocks of the country but in the backblocks of the world. But, symbolically, it was a purchase of some historical importance. This, 1876, was the year of the abolition of provincial government; pressures from the large landowners were henceforth to be disseminated and a vigorous band of politicians (Sir George Grey, Donald Reid, George Rolleston, John Williamson, John Ballance, James McKenzie) campaigned with zeal for the replacement of large estates by small farms. The depression of the sixties was over: the greater depression of the eighties was not foreseen. The country was filling with assisted immigrants (twenty-five thousand seven hundred in Canterbury alone between 1870 and 1879), and they looked to the small farmer for sustenance. The country, in fact, has been looking to the small farmer ever since. Canterbury could not live on its wool and was experimenting with wheat. A hard-working man on fifty acres might be a small national asset but when the efforts of all such men became aggregated a mighty potential resulted.

My grandfather probably never saw himself as a unit in a march but he probably experienced the magic of acquisition. When has man not hungered for a small portion of the earth's surface?

In 1876 the poor man, always fearful of the threat of charitable aid, had limited alternatives. He could in a small way, buy and sell, could barter, could command a wage or have the right to a small portion of land. This last was the precious choice. It was the only one with an element of security in it. Those who bought fifty acres in 1876 were rarely speculators. They sank their roots in the soil they owned, drew on its resources and were often content to be there at the end.

How could fifty acres support nine people? Yet in hundreds of cases fifty acres did. Ten acres for sheep, with wool to sell and never a shortage of mutton on the table. Ten acres for the horses and the cows, with milk, cream, butter and cheese. Twenty acres for wheat, a discovery almost as important to Canterbury as Gabriel's Gully was to Otago. (In the twelve year period following 1870 the Canterbury acreage of wheat rose from forty-six thousand to two hundred and forty-nine thousand.) It would be harvested on the small farm with scythe or sickle and the sheaves would be tied by hand. (Take two strands of wheat of a few straws each, twist and lock the ears, gather the wheat on the ground with a foot, bind each sheaf with the prepared straws, twist and bury the ends under the bands.) There was an artistry in this – a rhythm of motion, each sheaf taking only a few seconds.

The threshing was done with a flail. Milling was more difficult. Millers were expensive. Handmills were laborious. Somehow the flour was produced and the winter's bread was guaranteed.

Also on the fifty acres would be a few fruit trees and a vegetable garden and any farmer of enterprise would have periodic access to poultry, bush pigeons, rabbits, trout and ducks.

Mistress of the *ménage*, turning it from a house into a home was my indomitable grandmother. She had arrived in the *Zealandia* in 1858 along with her sisters and brothers (Foleys), the latter being the pioneers of vaudeville in New Zealand. She was soft-spoken with an Irish lilt and a confidence in it which carried her serenely along among her clutter of vigorous males. Though strongly Protestant she had been educated in a Dublin convent, so the family had been told, and this could well have been true for she never denied it.

The hard life of the pioneer woman has often been told but the emphasis has been on the episodic mischance or disaster. More wearing was the relentless toil of the endless days. My grandmother ran her boarding house, was mother to a large family, and had eleven confinements, all in Pleasant Valley without benefit of a doctor or a trained midwife. She nursed all the family through their illnesses, one of which ended fatally in a few months and another at twenty-two years. Before the Pleasant Valley school opened in 1875 she conducted a private school in her home. The hours were nine to twelve, five days a week, the syllabus was the three R's, eligible pupils were those who were illiterate and within walking distance, and the fees were nil. My father learned to read and write from his mother as I did from mine.

There are a number of stories of her strength and her endurance but they are not repeated here for though their basis was probably grounded in fact the later embellishments have increased the drama and marred the credibility.

Such were my paternal grandparents: pioneers, peasants, tireless workers in a raw land, persons of integrity and charity, grand people. Recently, a genealogist in Chester has tried to trace the earlier origins of my grandfather. He turned up several William Bennetts most of whom seemed to have been agricultural labourers and none of whom was likely to have been living in 1850 in a two storeyed house in the city of Chester. It matters little. The genes have come through whatever their origin.

My father left the crowded home at the age of sixteen defying his parents. This was in 1880, on the eve of the grim depression, second only in its misery to that of the 1930s. It was a calamitous time for a young manual worker to go forth to seek his fortune. All through his life he was to speak bitterly of the hungry eighties. Against the masses of unemployed married men a youth had little chance. For a time he tramped with the swaggers living off the back country station owners. Then he was employed as a cook's assistant in a shearing shed. This was a positive achievement even though it was the very lowest rung of the ladder for one who aspired to be champion shearer of New Zealand. (He eventually became an excellent shearer and during one season in the Waikato he withstood all challengers and was given the title of national champion, more through public agreement than through success in any controlled competition.) Most of his wandering years were spent in the North Island. He worked intermittently on the main trunk railway. He has described the pick and shovel gang and behind them the two lines of sitting men waiting for the occasional vacancy through sickness, accident or the foreman's displeasure. Once he tendered successfully for a large contract. For six months he fed and paid his gang and when the final balance sheet was drawn he had made a total profit of one pound. Yet this was the economic essence of the life of thousands – food and shelter, shelter and food in unstable periods of a few days at a time.

So through the anxious years till the better times of the mid-nineties he traded his labour and if he had little money he had received valuable experience. At the age of thirty he was back in Canterbury, a rough tough ranger of the backblocks. He looked around and found a job, worked it out and found another. But this was a road he had trodden too often. He was ready to exploit any new opportunity. And suddenly the opportunity came.

Meanwhile in Christchurch lived my other grandfather and the two stood in droll contrast. 'You in your small corner and I in mine.' James Harrow was a man of many interests and many crafts. Born in London (the birthplace of his ancestors as far back as he knew) in 1841, he was apprenticed as a brass moulder which seemed to be the key to unlock many talents. He became a gold and silver engraver, a gold beater and a designer of coloured lead-light windows. At times he made whips for coaches, then he was a coachsmith, a blacksmith, a policeman and a plumber. He was always improvising and inventing. He taught me how to make woodcarving tools out of umbrella ribs. He is said to have invented the kerosene pump but did not protect it by patent rights.

He who has lived in London always has a tale to tell. He remembered (being then eleven) the death of the Duke of Wellington. He worked at one stage in the laboratory of Michael Faraday whom he described as a kindly man. Once he was discovered by Faraday sleeping at his bench. Faraday gently woke him and suggested he get on with his work. He also worked for Lord Armstrong of the Vickers Armstrong Company. He played in the band that welcomed Garibaldi to London. He remembered Dr Barnado and also a lecture in a Wesleyan chapel in Woodgreen from a liberated slave named Josiah Henson who was supposed to be the original Uncle Tom.

Despite his inventiveness he was exasperatingly slow and cautious. And certainly time was kindly to him and his kin. He died at ninety-nine. My mother, despite her infirmity, lived till she was eighty-six. Her younger brother James who has retired to England is, in 1976, at the time of writing, robust and alert at the age of one hundred and nine. I once asked my grandfather about his boyhood life in London. He told a long narrative in which his father had introduced him to a visitor as the worst boy in London. To my grandfather the climax was in the visitor's comment that he had met many bad boys in London and that he considered it a privilege to meet the worst. To me the climax was in his added comment: 'I can't remember that man's name. But he was a great friend of my father and was often at our place. He had a bad limp. He had lost a leg at Waterloo.'

Then for obscure reasons in 1879 he with his wife, six children and a maid sailed for New Zealand in the *Piako* of one thousand tons. He paid one hundred and two pounds and ten shillings passage money for the nine persons. The first two nights in Christchurch were spent in the immigration barracks at Addington. He too was facing what was going to be the hungry eighties and the times were wrong for an aspiring goldsmith. After nine months the whole family returned to London. Within two years they were all back in Christchurch. He could no longer afford to choose his skills and the one most likely to succeed in those austere days was plumbing. So he became a plumber and his business in Gloucester Street was carried on through three generations for eighty years. Being a good plumber he made a fair living but his interests were elsewhere. He read widely – religion, fiction and science – and spent considerable leisure with his telescope and microscope.

The tap-tap-tap of the goldsmith's hammer in Christchurch had its counterpart in the wedge and maul of Pleasant Valley; and the rain would be thwarted by an umbrella in one place and a sack over the head in another. William Bennett would no more have read what James Harrow read than he would have read teacups. He claimed in fact to have read only one book in his life (*Uncle Tom's Cabin*), and he was put off books for ever because one character, Simon Legree, who should have been shot in the first chapter, was allowed to persist to the end.

Each grandfather jealously guarded his money. James Harrow kept his in the Savings Bank where interest was low but the security high. He once withdrew three hundred pounds as deposit for the purchase of the whole of the present residential part of the Cashmere Hills. After a week-end of agonized deliberation he put it back and ultimately invested it in two cottages in King Street, in one of which I was born. William Bennett, on the other hand, kept his savings under his bed, where they got no interest but were always available. They were also much safer than might appear. No burglar could approach without a vociferous challenge from the dogs, another challenge in the yard from one or more suspicious males, a traverse through the kitchen where my grandmother would be on guard and then into the bedroom itself where was a shotgun and a locked seachest.

James Harrow's wife was, in my recollection, a kindly person but a shadowy personality. She was in continued ill-health (a diabetic in the grim pre-insulin days) and she died about 1913. Her eldest daughter, Rose, was fifteen when she first arrived in Christchurch. She developed into a person of charm – slim, petite, clear skinned and golden haired. There were many men in the next decade who tried to persuade her to change her name. She was well read, a pianist and organist, an accomplished needlewoman and adept at leather work. She established her own dressmaking business in Colombo Street approximately where Minson's establishment now is.

And there she was, the successful business-woman, when she met William Bennett. It seemed the most unlikely of associations – the delicate flower from London and a rugged bit of undergrowth from South Canterbury. Its basis was unknown, for they would never talk of it, but it almost certainly leaned heavily on the fact that they both became deeply committed Christians, rigid in their belief in the authenticity of the Bible and its authority to command their lives. Most likely she converted him. Or perhaps someone else did and her interest was roused. For him it was an almost incredible change. Certainly his life in the shearing sheds had no spiritual content. Of the rest, which is their private story, only the facts survive. They became engaged. My father, adjusting to 'settling down', bought his father's farm of fifty acres at Pleasant Valley. His father moved to a new property of two hundred and three acres at Fairfield taking with him four rooms of the old house. My mother went to Pleasant Valley and apparently approved. They were married in Christchurch and he in the meanwhile had furnished the house. As they journeyed down he said 'I have a nice surprise for you in the front room'. She could think only of a piece of antique furniture and wondered where he had got it. The incident illustrated the differences in their two cultures. The front room floor was covered from wall to wall with drying walnuts.

At the end of a year I was born and about the same time there occurred the first symptoms of rheumatoid arthritis. It was crippling and alarming and the widely held belief at the time was that it was due to the damp. In Pleasant Valley, heavily bushed, with probably a faulty house and a high water table as proved by the farmer's only water supply coming from a bricklined well, recovery was unlikely. So the farm was sold to Joseph Robinson and my father bought his new farm at Woodbury.

It is appropriate to add a footnote to each of these three farms with four ownerships by two people. The Pleasant Valley farm is still owned by a member of the Robinson family though no one any longer lives there. There are two arable paddocks, some massed macrocarpas on the site of the house, and, on the hillside, walnut trees, a group of sycamores, a spreading poplar, blue gums and hazel nuts – planted by my grandmother about the same time as similar trees were planted in Hagley Park and, now, just as mighty and magnificent. This was the territory of my ancestors and here I must have lived for my first eighteen months. I have been back recently but the only ghost there now is that of my mother. In her youth London had been wide open. Now she was anchored in a prison of isolation on the very rim of the world. The bell birds in the tree tops had replaced the Bow Bells within whose sound she had been born. The unremitting London traffic had yielded to the magpies quarrelling in the pines. Her joints were stiffening, the pain increasing, the baby grew heavier, the farm was small and the times were hard. On the road an occasional dray would pass. Outside the house was a tall dark man struggling with a team. Where the house once stood is now a confusion of macrocarpas. The other four rooms, papered with newspapers of about 1872, which were my parents' first home (and mine), still exist on the Four Peaks farm of the present owner. They house hay and chaff which tend to keep the walls standing.

Fairfield remained in my grandfather's possession for about twenty years and then he sold it and retired to Timaru. His family had scattered, usually on hardy missions. Two went to the Boer War; another was wounded on the Somme. Like their father they were restless, energetic and tireless workers. Despite the depression, their work potential was such that they were never unemployed. All their days were long days. I remember my grandfather appearing every morning at his back door and yelling across 'Five o'clock Henry. Get up Henry.' This was imitated by a tame magpie which was one of the many curiosities of the place. The magpie would sometimes shriek at Henry that it was five o'clock when it was only four. Henry, permitted to ignore one summons, often ignored both. The magpie was threatened, and when it tried to persuade Henry that it was five o'clock when it was only three, this became its swan song and it departed this life.

Despite their toughness they had a rough sympathy with the unfortunate. The story of Murphy (a name of convenience) comes to mind. He was an arthritic cripple living alone in his little hut deep down in the gully. He once had ten acres of oats in stook. Night and morning he and his dray made their tortured way up the hill where he added another drayful to the stack in a futile race against the winter rains. One early afternoon a homing harvesting gang with the usual two drays and five men, three of them being Bennett brothers, was passing. Those in the first dray threw open the gate and began to load. The others followed. There was no plan, no discussion. For three hours there was at least one sheaf in the air all the time. In the cool of the evening Murphy came zigzagging up the hill. What he thought was never known. What he saw was his paddock, clean and bare except for two stacks in the centre, expertly built and weighted down. The gate was closed and no one was in sight. He never knew the truth, but everyone else did, for there had been witnesses. He was not an intellectual, and he firmly believed in spirits good and bad and confidently used them when confronted with a mystery. He asserted as time went by that the miracle in his paddock had been effected by the good spirits, namely by the angels. In time he came to believe this. Whenever he could be enticed into the Arowhenua hotel (not a difficult task) and plied with free whisky (even less difficult) he would reach the imaginative heights of having seen the blessed angels flitting about the paddock with a sheaf under each arm. The audience was always greatly entertained, not so much at the gullibility of Murphy as at the incongruity of the Bennett brothers being mistaken for angels.

After seven or eight years on the Woodbury farm my parents were forced to acknowledge some awkward truths. The rheumatoid arthritis was steadily getting worse, Rotorua notwithstanding, and there were now four boys and hope of a daughter had to be abandoned. With the increased family (even though the third boy was being brought up by his grandmother at Fairfield) my father could no longer combine the duties of house and farm. Domestic help was not available. Also Woodbury was damp or was presumed to be. A larger home, nearer to schools and to a civilized centre, a home with perhaps a little elegance, in deference to my mother, then became the new objective. So the farm was sold to a local farmer, Mr Rice who, with his descendants, has occupied it for over sixty years. The house at the end of Rice's Road still exists though it is now altered beyond recognition. The saplings have become mighty giants. The creek babbles on but the flax has gone. The stables are full of machinery where once were the horses, horse covers and chaff. Not only is there no white towel over the gate but the gate has vanished along with the duckpond and the pyramid of stones.

So we left Woodbury, insecure wanderers in search of a farm. There were transit camps with relatives in Christchurch and Timaru while my father went on searching. Finally in 1907 he led us to our new home at Fairview, six miles west of Timaru.

3

School Bells

There were three significant schools: Fairview, Timaru Boys' High and the Medical School, representing primary, secondary and university education. But these were preceded by three others, deserving only a minor tick statistically and no tick at all educationally.

The first was the Sydenham school in Christchurch. I was probably five, my brother four. Our mother was in Rotorua and we were in the care of her sister, the most indulgent of aunts. We revelled in our introduction to the great city. Our bedroom faced east, and at dawn we would see the light straining at the sky and streaming through the notched skyline of the hills. With this went the chorus of the roosters fighting it out, suburb by suburb. Then in the full day came the water carts in the dusty streets and council drays collecting manure till the firebell rang and the horses would be turned out to gallop back to the station. Picnics were by double-decker trams to Sumner or by train to Lyttelton from where we sometimes walked to Corsair Bay. There was one occasion when a Health Inspector was reported to be making a house-to-house survey in Milton Street and my aunt rushed to turn on all the taps and sent me flying down the street to warn the neighbours. The Health Inspectors were perhaps more feared than the police for they aimed at property. The standard of sanitation required rested with them. If a property owner did not comply, his property could be destroyed. By modern standards they were poorly informed, given to gross errors of judgement and were dangerously autocratic. Even I, racing to thwart them, felt the thrill of striking a small blow for what I felt was justice.

Fascinating, too, were the shops, especially those where we spent our weekly pocket money of a penny each (sometimes withheld because of poor conduct). Our favourite purchase was a lolly bird's nest with four eggs, which seemed to be the pick of the market. But balanced against such trivia were the horse-drawn funerals. Almost daily they would come down Colombo Street and turn into Milton Street on their way to Spreydon cemetery. Invariably my brother and I would fall in behind the mourners marching four abreast. We would conduct ourselves with great decorum even to and from the graveside. Probably we were many times erroneously placed in the family tree of the deceased and commended for our fortitude in bereavement. Our motive was utterly obscure.

All this is better remembered than my few weeks at the Sydenham school where I probably lost all identity in the mass. J. P. Morrison, in her *Evolution of a City* (Christchurch, Christchurch City Council, 1948), describes the Sydenham school of that time:

> Teachers struggled with classes of 90 pupils. Small children learnt their alphabet and read school primers, used copy-books for a set style of hand-writing, copied their drawings from the teacher's black-board model and spent hours being drilled in multiplication tables.

This would have held little interest for one who could read and write. The main incident I remember was in the playground where I discovered my brother trying to ward off a bully twice his size. I went to his assistance but we lacked a battle plan, attacked in turn and got laid out in turn.

Yet we had a great regard for our teacher. (She had probably intervened in some bullying episode.) She was Miss Adams of the Luke Adams Pottery works in Colombo Street. We visited her to say goodbye and she gave us a box of small ornamental bricks. She said she expected us to grow up to be very good boys and she was going to watch our future with very great interest. (About forty years later when she and I were professionally involved she denied all previous knowledge of me.)

The Sydenham school made little impact on us and we reciprocated. We were a couple of country urchins, probably compassionately enrolled because of an invalid mother and a harassed aunt. Yet, nearly half a century later I was invited, as an old boy, to some anniversary of the school. At least the records were exemplary.

Then from the high adventures of Christchurch we went back to the placid familiarity of Woodbury: the creek and the flax, the old chaff mattress, the animals, the makeshift toys, the winter frosts outlining the enormous spider webs on the gorse bushes. My mother was back home apparently as incapable of walking as before. There was an emotional reunion even though I knew she would exact from me far more than my kindly aunt had done.

Education in those days was a desirable acquisition, but like butter on the bread was not essential. Even my father's schooldays preceded the legislation of 1877 which made education free, secular and compulsory. But a sociological advance often has to wait twenty five years before it is accepted publicly. At the beginning of this century there was still much apathy regarding schooling, and truant officers were almost as active then as parent-teacher associations are today. Although the inevitable stubborn

31

fringe claimed that education threatened their young with eye strain or brain fever, or loss of freedom or wrong doctrination, the majority of the people were convinced of the efficacy of the three R's. Yet only some of these could find any merit in secondary education. Unnecessary knowledge was a burdensome weight, it was no asset to those seeking a manual job, and its power to develop latent personalities was little known.

I was not enrolled at the Woodbury school till I was eight. This was not due to parental indifference but because I was essential at home. I think my mother must have tried to offset this by making herself my teacher, and certainly in the matter of reading she had brought us far ahead of the average at that age. My father, who liked to see in me a pocket edition of himself and his father with all the rough spots showing, had a simple formula for my education. 'First you must learn to swim, ride and shoot. Then you can take up your books.'

One by one I satisfied these prerequisites. The first was swimming, which was learnt in our flax-girt creek meandering through its deep pools and rapid shallows. We usually crossed it on a tree trunk fallen over a deep but narrow pool. This pool was one terminal of a U-bend and the returning arm was not far away. Between the two my father had dug a ditch and whenever my mother (or anyone else) had a desire for trout he would drop in some boards at the outlet of the pool and flood the water across country. This drained the chain or so of the U-bend leaving a number of trout flapping in shallow pools. He would then go along selecting the prime ones. I have several angling friends who describe this method of fishing as the lowest imaginable. But they miss the point. He was not fishing. He was getting trout for my mother.

One day he crossed over the pool then turned to watch me following. When I was half way across, swaying with arms extended he put his foot on the tree trunk and rolled it. I had hardly time to yell before I was submerged. As I came up he shouted, 'You've got to learn to swim. Now's the time.' It was certainly the time if survival was to be part of it. Desperately I splashed out and when I reached the bank he helped me out. 'Now you can swim,' he informed me. I was not sure. That afternoon I went back, stripped off and conducted some experiments. Finally I swam the pool from side to side. There was no doubt that, as usual, he was right. I could swim. Then came riding. On Sunday he and I were returning from a service in Geraldine when there was a confrontation, with one of our mares (and foal) bound for freedom. My father, hurrying to get home to my mother, turned the mare round, improvised a halter, mounted me and drove off. On the beast's back my legs stuck out at right angles and had I worn spurs I could not have used them. A struggle for supremacy between these two six-year-olds ensued and the horse won, stopping and feeding where it liked. Its dawdling foal was obviously a delinquent.

So we came funereally to Woodbury, which should have been as desolate as an unmanned station on the moon. Instead round the closed store were nearly a dozen local youths blue-suited, celluloid-collared and red-faced, all ripe for diversion which in its richest form might involve the passing of several girls ready to reciprocate in an exciting interchange of banter. Instead, on this occasion I hove into view and they adopted me as a substitute. It pleased them to regard me as a jockey of renown, engaged in a tense struggle as I rounded into the straight. They shouted advice, laid bets on me, advocated a freer use of the whip. I stared ahead, unseeing, unhearing, uncompromising, making a claim to dignity as preposterous as that of a chimp on the back of a circus pony.

By mid-afternoon I reached home and slid off the horse's back. With great difficulty I approximated my legs. My father observed, 'Taken you a long time'. I dared not tell him I had lost the foal. But I did not know the ways of mares and foals. That evening I saw them grazing together by the side of the house.

My first lesson in shooting was for some years my last, so well did it instruct me in the principles of caution. Once again I was staying with my grandparents at Fairfield. One day the cry went up that there was a hawk hovering over some chickens. My grandfather strode out with the gun but the hawk was now out of range. He laid the gun down on the crest of the hill with the barrel projecting into mid-air above the slope. He then went down the hill. Ten minutes later he trudged back, his course being in the same projection as the barrel of the gun. In the meantime I, confident of his absence, was examining the gun. Suddenly there was a flash and a roar. My grandfather dropped flat. His hat had been blown off his head and a few pellets had perforated it. Then he was on his feet bellowing like a bull and making for me. But I was on the flat and my legs were terror-fired. My grandmother came running, swept me into the shelter of her skirts and hustled me to a back room. Into the house he came, still bellowing, but he could not get beyond her firm defence. It was three days before we met again. Each refused to be aware of the other, and in this role he quite outshone me. I could not understand my uncles' tolerance. They were curiously urbane and almost regarded the whole dreadful business with amusement. They would ruffle my hair and say 'Well, young codger, what have you been up to today?' Apparently they had a certain admiration for my marksmanship. This, I suppose, was justified. William Tell had achieved world-wide fame for doing no better despite his advantage of a co-operative partner.

Woodbury School drew me like a magnet. At last I had a status in the world which was not imaginative. Every morning I donned importance and strode forth slamming the gate behind me, slashing at thistles with a stick, kicking puffballs out of my path, warming to the admiration of an imaginary audience. Unaware of the tedious logic of Euclid, I knew that the two sides of a triangle were greater than the third. So I often made a beeline for Woodbury by cutting diagonally across the stony paddock of a neighbour. Occasionally he would appear, and from afar off would shout at me unintelligibly and yet with menace. As a result I usually kept to the highway for the next few days. But there was never any confrontation. His name, appropriately enough, was Barker.

There were two rooms to the school. The junior room was a sounding stage for a racket of shrill voices and was under the nominal control of a distracted young lady who believed strongly, but disastrously, in persuasion and coercion. The senior room was known to be a fearsome place given to tortures and brutality and even, so it was whispered in the lower school, to an occasional disappearance. Every morning a senior boy (a survivor) would march into the playground, lick his finger, hold it upright and make a note. A modern method, explained my father, of revealing the direction of the wind. The old method of course was to look at the trees.

I remember nothing of the teaching. Much of it had to do with the laboured mechanics of the alphabet and with learning to write. Also we spent long periods drawing shapes like cuphooks, apparently in the interests of calligraphy. I ignored all this and began to fill in the blank periods with the dangerous diversion of day-dreaming.

The life of the school centred round the playgrounds, one for the boys and one for the girls. The latter must also have been open to boys in the primers, for we were often in contact, and in conflict, with the girls. Usually the primer boys stuck together, mainly because no one else could be bothered with them. We were a boisterous bunch, racing and chasing with shrill noise and no purpose. All of us were probably meeting in gregarious and exciting equality for the first time.

We had our games. A favourite was 'Monkey', where the contestant climbed one of the fir trees along one side of the ground (still there at the present day) and did a grand traverse of as many trees as possible. It was characterized by noise, boasting, cheating and an occasional sprained wrist. There was cockfighting in which each of two players, mounted pick-a-back, tried to resist dislodgement. Disputed ownership of any article was automatically resolved into a wrestling match. At times we would make a raid on the girls, who would flee for the safety of the senior

34

playground. The object was to prevent their reaching this sanctuary, to trip them up, roll them on the grass, savour their fear, and then stride off triumphant in masculinity.

One day in one of these sorties a girl was sent flying and landed on her back. I had had no part in this and was merely a spectator. But it was no place for spectators for the wretched girl had, in dressing that morning, overlooked the most vital garment, and I had my first lesson in female anatomy. It was only a passing glimpse and all it aroused in me was a surge of incredulity. I had had no idea that anyone could be so deformed, so maimed by such a gross deviation from the norm and yet be so brave about it. Apparently with girls you never could tell. I did not chase them again.

We arrived at school singly, but those who lived down the Peel Forest Road started for home in a body. We dawdled through Woodbury at a pace which meant that most of the time we were stationary. The first check-point was the store, selling everything from patent medicines to horse collars. It was a place of exotic odours. He who had a pretext for entering the store was considered lucky. A few like me with no older family representative at the school would march in boldly and demand the family mail and would be genuinely surprised if there was any. On the opposite corner of the cross-roads was the blacksmith's where it was fascinating to stand at the door and dangerous to go any further. Inside were pungent fumes, flying sparks, a fearsome roaring at the touch of the bellows, the clang of steel and enormous horses standing on three legs. The blacksmith, blue-shirted and leather aproned, strode fearlessly about. At times he would lunge towards us with a red-hot bar and we would scatter, but like flies disturbed on a honey pot, would soon be back. He had no malevolence towards us but it heightened the illusion to pretend that he had. At times he would treat us to snippets of worldly wisdom which was generous in so mighty a man. He said we were an idle lot of little crawlers, that we were lucky to be going to school and that the country was spending more on us than it could afford. We probably gave him more attention than we gave our teachers. We obediently departed at his dismissal 'Now get home you lazy little devils and do some work'. And that was Woodbury, except for a house or two. We shunned only the fishman. He was an old man who came round once a week and under the seat in his trap were a couple of boxes of fish which he sold from door to door. He was the subject of the ugliest rumours. Several boys last seen talking to him had never been seen again and in each instance fish was cheap and plentiful the next week. I suppose we did not believe it, but belief and caution are different things and if the evil old man was about we herded together and hurried past. None of us suspected that the wise old man may have started the rumour.

A mile past Woodbury I left the gang and went down a side road. I plodded on, pausing only for matters of real interest and my average pace was a mile an hour. I was ever in trouble at home for late arrival. Education at school did not mean emancipation at home. I was supposed to contribute to the evening bustle that closed the day. A dreary road to the modern motorist (as I have recently verified) but an absorbing road to an eight-year-old pedestrian. Fences, ditches, hedgerows, rabbits, plant life and an occasional daring trespass into a neighbour's, all demanded interest and time. 'At last you're home,' my mother would say wearily. 'What have you been doing?'

One afternoon our scrubby little gang was at the door of the forge where our local Vulcan was shoeing a draught. He dropped the hoof and came towards us.

'Which of you is young Bennett? Come here boy.' This was frightening. I stepped out.

'Can you give a message to your father?'

'Yes.'

'Tell him Dick Seddon's dead. Go on, say it.'

'Dick Seddon's dead.'

'Now don't forget. Dick Seddon's dead.'

I reached home. My father was in the kitchen stoking the range with slabs of wood. Without looking round he said, 'You're late again. What's the excuse this time?'

'Dick Seddon's dead.'

He straightened up and looked at me with some amusement. 'And what do you know about Dick Seddon?'

'Nothing – except that he's dead.'

'Who told you?' he asked sharply.

I described the circumstances. The blacksmith was a political friend incapable of bogus messages. My father slammed up the door of the firebox and went off to my mother. I heard them discussing it, sadly, late into the night.

Then the farm was sold and the Woodbury adventure was over. I have forgotten all I was ever taught there but I have not forgotten all I learned. On leaving, the world was a wider place. Over fifty years later I was invited to an anniversary. Within the last year I have been back. There is a new school of course. There are now no thumbscrews or treadmills in the senior room. It was perhaps appropriate that I should be asked to address the junior school. It was not a successful address for I started by telling them how long ago I had been to the school and this left them completely bewildered. But they thanked me at the end in a

·pretty chorus. Nice kids. Nicer than their great-grandparents as I remember them.

The third of the transient schools was the Timaru Main School. While my father was cautiously buying a farm we lived with an aunt at the lower end of North Street and it was inevitable that my brother and I should be sent up the road to school. Nothing is now remembered of that very short period except one traumatic incident. I was in one of the lower standards in a great room full of strange children. The only lesson I remember was arithmetic and now in retrospect it seemed to fill all day and every day. The only person I remember was the teacher. She was above average height and was proportionately weighty, and was all curves without seductiveness. She threw her head and shoulders back and her bosom advanced like the prow of a war canoe. Her voice was loud and harsh and lacked any feminine overtones. In her hand she carried continually a black leather strap, about an inch wide and a quarter of an inch thick.

All the trouble centred round what was called (I think) long multiplication where a three-figured number had to be multiplied by a two-figured number. The method had never been explained to me. Her procedure was to write the two numbers on the board and then while the class was scratching out answers on their slates she would move down and through the class looking over shoulders. Then with a slap of the strap on a desk she would call the class to attention and demand the answer from some unfortunate. If he were wrong he would be ordered out to the front. Then she would ask another pupil. Eventually a correct answer would be given. 'Hands up those who got it right.' A forest of hands would go up, mine included. She would then proceed to strap those at the front, one, two or three cuts, after which, fighting their tears they would sink back into their places, having presumably been put on the right road for becoming better mathematicians. I am not certain now as to all the qualifications for the strap, but it was in use all through all lessons.

She terrified me and at last I approached her after school.

'Please Miss, I've never been shown how to do these sums.'

'Well you had better find out pretty soon or you'll be in trouble.' And she walked away.

Inevitably there had to be a crisis. One day she set a sum and then began roaming through the class. From well behind me I heard her approve the right answer. Hastily I rubbed out the numbers I had guessed, wrote in the right ones and raised my hand. But she had moved up just behind me. I was marched out to the front and got three cuts on each hand, one lot presumably because I was ignorant and the other because I pretended not to be.

37

That evening, the pain having gone, but the rage remaining, a gulp betrayed me.

'What's the matter, son?' my father asked.

'Nothing.'

'Come on. What's it all about?'

I poured it out, breaking down in the process. He asked questions. Then he said:

'Well now, about those sums first.' He got a pencil and paper. 'This is how you do it.' It was so simple. Multiply the first number by each of the other figures in turn being careful to put them in the right places and then add them all up.

'Is that all you do?'

'That's all. Now here are some sums. You do them while I'm out.'

'Where are you going?'

'Just out.'

When he came back the sums were all done and at least half of them were right which meant that at last technique was taking over from guesswork.

'She'll get a surprise tomorrow,' I said.

'No she won't. She won't even be surprised that you're not there. You're not going back to that school.'

Corporal punishment is among the most persistent of the social evils. Though the foundations on which it once stood – precedent, tradition, Solomon, the Bible, desperation, common sense, political approval – have all been toppled, it still persists, usually in secondary schools where it is nurtured by a small chauvinistic group of masters and old boys. On the subject the clichés abound. 'There is no other way of reaching the hard core of the defiant ones' (masters); 'the present generation should learn to take it as we did' (old boys); 'at all costs discipline must be preserved' (Board); none of these have probed the difficult depths of reason to determine what is the purpose of punishment. It is easier to stand up with a cane than to sit down with a problem. Corporal punishment combines the elements of revenge for the past and the deterrent of fear in the future which are two of the lowest motives for any punishment. It may stop the act but it increases the enmity and drives it dangerously underground. The apologists have their patter, 'This hurts me more than it hurts you,' which almost invariably is a lie. 'If you are brave it doesn't hurt.' This is another lie. It hurts like hell. Pain is second only to touch in the chronological evolution of the human nervous system and is a fearsome stimulus to self-defence. The little group of scourgers know nothing of neurology nor how they are prostituting a physiological function for a punitive purpose. The torture of political prisoners and the corporal punishment of educational prisoners are but variants of the same process.

My Amazon of the Timaru Main School was a sadist who probably stood in very good repute with the headmaster, the Board and herself. All would have applauded her great competence in the matter of discipline. Her cringing class was powerless. Every day by means of the strap she made them fear the more the subject she was supposed to teach. Yet only two years before, Mr Bishop S.M., in fining a teacher for strapping a girl of thirteen, said, 'It seemed absurd for a teacher to come into court and say he could teach spelling only by use of the strap.' (See *Lyttelton Times*, 7 June 1905.)

Then came Fairview School. It was typical of the many country schools of the time, all roughly comparable in function and purpose. These schools were administered by the Canterbury Education Board with funds supplied by the Department of Education. Each Board was elected by the various local school committees which also selected the teachers and normally supervised the maintenance of the school. As has been implied, education particularly in the primary schools did not rank high in the country's culture. The teachers suffered proportionately. As confirmed by all later historians they were (especially in the smaller schools) ill-trained and ill-paid. Yet they were enormously important for within the school walls they had an almost complete autonomy. The Department supplied a syllabus but it was too wide to have any depth. The school committee dealt only with complaints and isolated incidents. Twice a year the Inspector came for half a day. The date was always known and our fingernails would be clean and our boots polished. He (in my day Mr Gow) would be hearty and affable, rustling through exercise books, asking questions and then going off to lunch with the teacher and, according to her, leaving an assurance that he was very pleased with us all. The next day the teacher would take over the controls again and the school would chug off on the rails of routine.

The desire to write of the Fairview school is partly an historical compulsion. Those who attended such schools in the first decade of the century have left little on record. Now if anything is to be added from first hand sources there is little time to spare.

Firstly then as to the setting. The school was in a squarish uneven paddock of four acres with a deep dray track crossing diagonally the entrance gates to the teacher's house. It was enclosed on all sides by a belt of firs. There were no other trees, shrubs or flowers. There were toilets deservedly hidden in the trees and a flagpole prominent in the open. It was our playground in the sense that it was the ground on which we played.

The school was a rectangular box with a small entrance porch at the narrow end whence opened the only door to the schoolroom. Inside on the right, high up near the ceiling, was a series of small windows framing the sky and effectively guarding against distraction but not against day-dreaming. The windows were manipulated by a brass hook on a long pole. Immediately inside the door on the other side was a table carrying a set of pigeon holes and on the wall was a telephone. This was the Fairview public Post Office. Halfway down the wall was a large open fireplace. Pause to consider the menace of fire. In the school there was no fire drill. The only exit was through the one door at the far end. The windows were too high to be escape routes. There seemed a curious indifference to fire at the time. The Fire Brigade Act was not passed till 1906 and was modified in 1907 and 1908. Yet in all the years I spent in the country I never remember any incident of a house on fire. Whether our home carried fire insurance I do not know, but I would be surprised if it did. My father always liked to see something for his money. I have of recent years reviewed at times the almost incredible situation at Woodbury where my mother was completely confined to an easy chair a few feet away from a wood-burning stove. If the kitchen had suddenly blazed her life would have depended on her very young son.

In the centre of the schoolroom was the teacher's desk with the blackboard on one side and the piano on the other. Beyond, jammed together were the forms (backless) and desks for the thirty to forty pupils. In a far corner was a large bookcase, dusty, almost empty. There was a cupboard near the door and a few maps scattered about, but these were decorative for I never remember anyone studying them. Presiding over it all was Miss Helen C. W. Johnston of Dunedin.

The illusion of a liberal primary education was founded on the many approved subjects in the teaching syllabus. This wide range seemed to be mainly for the benefit of the teacher. From it she could select subjects which she was competent to teach and at which her classes could work unattended. The school curriculum therefore depended on the teacher's whim though there were probably special obligations about reading and writing. The educational requirements were satisfied if the pupil 'took' for the appropriate time any item on the list, even if it were almost exclusively one of the more bizarre subjects, such as embroidery.

A day in the school would begin at nine a.m. when Miss Johnston would appear at the porch door and ring the handbell. We would follow her back and scramble to our places. At no stage in our school life was there any formality or drill. The first half hour or so was usually devoted to singing. The whole school from the tots to the teens formed a shrill choir.

There was no conductor other than Miss Johnston energetically thumping on the piano. Our repertoire revealed us to be a patriotic choir of sturdy little Imperialists. We swept through the British Isles with 'Rule Britannia', 'Scots Wha Hae', 'Men of Harlech' and 'The Dear Little Shamrock'. We then acknowledged the Maple Leaf our Emblem Dear and the need for God to Defend New Zealand. We also indulged in some of those quixotic compositions called rounds, the favourite being 'London's Burning'. These started melodiously enough but finished in chaos as the fire got out of control. Our most dramatic item was a spine tingling version of the Marseillaise. 'March on, march on,' we would sing as if addressing our bare and grubby feet. 'Death or victory'; at the top of our voices we scorned anything else, and in the paddock across the road my father's cows would look up in mild perplexity. We didn't understand it. But then we also didn't understand what 'Scots wha hae' would be in English nor where Harlech was.

The singing over, the problems of Miss Johnston began. Theoretically she had four primers and six standards. She could teach only one at a time and the other nine would have to be self-employed, but only within the range allowed by the syllabus. Actually there were never nine. She compacted the whole school up into blocks for ease of processing. One of these groups she would teach and for the rest would set tasks that required the minimum of supervision. At mid-morning there was a playtime of fifteen minutes during which we rushed about noisily and aimlessly. Then the bell went again and we settled down for another hour. Miss Johnston after such breaks would take another class and had employed the interval by setting certain tasks on the blackboard for the rest. The aim was to find something for everyone to do. This period was usually interrupted by the arrival of the postman, a tall swaggering type who would march in after one loud knock on the door, fling down his mailbag and pick up the empty one. He usually had a few banal words for the school, 'Get on with your work, don't mind me'. 'Lucky you are to get an education. We never got it.' 'Wait till you have to earn your living.' These liberties gave no pleasure to Miss Johnston as her manner plainly showed. But his presence there was official and he leaned heavily on it. In winter he collected his two hot bricks from the fireplace leaving two cold ones for the morrow. This exchange he effected at every school on his daily circuit.

At midday we had an hour for lunch which we ate in about ten minutes and after that resorted to play. There was no playground supervision of any sort and no facilities or equipment for sport of any kind. We were left to our own devices and the result was poor. In our few games more time was spent in quarrelling over the rules than in applying them. We had elaborate competitions with pocket knives based on a series of flips and tricks of increasing difficulty. All the boys had pocket knives as symbols of impending manhood and the prestige value of each was based not on the cutting blade but on the auxiliaries of corkscrew, tin opener, screwdriver, et cetera. Wherever we went we doggedly carried these futile weights. I once owned an unwieldy mass of ironware boasting no less than ten gadgets, one of which was a metal probe for extracting a stone from a horse's hoof. The occasion of course never arose but there was much satisfaction in knowing that if it ever did I was prepared. We fought, savagely and bare-fistedly. Never a week but two of these fights provided spectator excitement in the lunch hour. In nearly every instance the motive was to establish the courage of each contestant. If anyone suggested that A was afraid of B the matter had to be put to the test. It was possible to select two juniors, natural bland innocents, and by means of goading and taunting have them swinging wildly while they gulped back their sobs. It was as senseless as modern gang warfare or the logic of a medieval knight jousting with death in defence of something known as a lady's honour.

Even more reprehensible was our language. It was heavy with reference to sex and the excreta. Because of my home influence I contributed little to this yet I let it pass without protest. I was powerless beneath the tradition of conformity. All of the objectionable allusions were of course copied from adults. We were not aware of the bathos when eroticism was mimicked by those who had not yet reached puberty. The playground was never more than the arena for the conflicts of boys. Our right to the ground was the right of might. The girls, cynical and sulky, were in little groups among the trees. We played Cowboys and Indians, building elaborate forts with pine needles, but these could be demolished with a kick which was usually followed by a fight.

At one o'clock the bell rang again. Miss Johnston called a new class to the front. The rest of us became more or less self-employed. If we kept reasonably quiet and appeared to be industrious we were apparently being processed in the educational mill. At two thirty the primers noisily departed. Another hour, the longest of the school day, dragged its tortured length until Miss Johnston finished with her class and went to her postal pigeon holes. We crowded round waiting for mail which was usually no more than the *Timaru Herald*. Then out on the road, half went up and half went down and another school day was over.

I had good reason to remember our first football, for at the time I thought I had provided it. With dictatorial crudity I had imposed a levy of threepence each on all males over ten. It was not a popular appeal. The fund closed at two shillings. At this stage my father became involved. He took the money and came back from Timaru with a new, shiny, sweet-smelling rugby ball. I was amazed that they were so cheap. We had two glorious days pretending to be the 1905 All Blacks and then Miss Johnston demanded to see the ball and expressed deep displeasure that she she was not first consulted. She emphasized this by impounding the ball. Quivering with indignation I laid it all before my father. He sided with her. Politeness demanded that she should be aware of all school activities. But that evening I noticed him putting on his coat, and strolling over to the school. The next morning the ball was on the porch.

Before we had properly mastered the rules of rugby we challenged Adair, a neighbouring school. We paid dearly. Though it was a smaller school it had one indomitable player, Jack Hutton. He had had a mid-thigh amputation in infancy which marred his sporting career but did not destroy it. At the Timaru Boys' High School later he regularly won the high jump, many photos having proved that his two crutches and one leg were all off the ground at the one time. As captain of the Adair team he was devastating. He would lead a forward rush swinging his crutches wildly and the Fairview team would abandon the ball and scuttle for safety. Adair School was full of resources. For long it topped the bird egg collections. The county council paid threepence a dozen for eggs and once a month their representative would visit each school, inspect the filthy mass we turned out of our treacle tins, and write a voucher. Then he would bury the fragile eggs and fragment them by tramping. But, for some years, the Adair eggs were dug up again and resold, having first been hard boiled.

Every morning after our discordant tour of the Empire Miss Johnston set most of the school to the subjects which had, so to speak, an automatic drive. The favourite subjects were handwork, freehand drawing, silent reading and 'doing a composition', i.e. writing an essay.

These were items of schooling but not of education. Handwork for the girls meant what could be done with one needle, one thimble and one reel of cotton. For the boys it meant chip carving. It was performed on a standard article of a teatray – a kauri slab about sixteen inches by ten with a raised edge and two wooden handles (cost, two and sixpence). The design to be carved was determined by the carver. He invariably began with some intersecting circles, marked off the perimeter into six sections (approximately equal), connected some of these to the centre, added a few frills and eventually arrived at an incomprehensible mesh of ellipses. Miss Johnston took no interest in them and gave no instruction. Periodically we would ask her to sharpen our chip knives which she always did, giving the blade a few gentle ineffectual strokes as if she were fondling a kitten. Yet to her it was a valued educational tranquillizer ('You boys in the back seats, stop that noise. Get out your carving'). The trays were proudly exhibited at the school break-up and were always approved by the parents who felt that some aesthetic resources had thereby been tapped. The trays in fact were an abomination. Kauri which is one of the noblest creations should never be so mutilated. They could function as teatrays only if they were upside down. Afternoon tea in Fairview required no grace of trays. It was taken off a corner of the kitchen table cleared for the purpose or else from a basket and billy out in the paddock.

Freehand drawing was an innocuous method of marking off another educational period. Miss Johnston would set up a stark bit of still life – a bottle, a cup, a box – and with timid pencil and confident rubber we would transform the white page into a smeared mess. There was no instruction. We had never heard of perspective.

The upper classes could always be reduced to some orderliness by making them 'do a composition'. Though the subjects were usually homely I always had to treat them with discretion. What I did in the holidays could hardly be answered by a reference to my father, who set the daily work load; nor could I say that my day at the show was mainly spent crawling under the tent flaps of the side shows; nor could an essay on my favourite pet reveal my liking for chocolate fish.

Then came silent reading. It was not a popular subject for there was little to read. The *School Journal* began in 1907 and I was a foundation subscriber. It was absorbing for half an hour of every month. Beyond was the boredom of inactivity. I had arrived at the school without any credentials and Miss Johnston accepted my word that I was in Standard Three which was debatable (my brother who was in Primer Two declared he was in Standard Two and this brought him uncomfortably close). Miss Johnston commended my reading and deplored my arithmetic and turned me loose in the school to find my own level like everyone else. I soon improved the arithmetic. I searched the school for something to read and seemed destined to an education career restricted to carving teatrays or trying to make the two sides of a teapot symmetrical. 'Read the daily paper,' Miss Johnston kept imploring us, which was all she could do to enlighten us on the subjects of geography, history and civic affairs.

Then suddenly, a connected series of casual events built up into a situation which – I use the phrase with considered restraint – changed my life. It began with the man, unknown to me, whose donation (legacy?) to the Timaru Boys' High School Library was of such an order that the Board decided to replace and dump all the old books. Somehow my father, who had just become chairman of the local school committee, heard of this and he went to Timaru in a dray with a five pound note and came back with two or three hundred dog-eared volumes and piled them in the big bookcase in the far corner of the schoolroom. In this corner I settled intent on a career of silent reading. Miss Johnston seemed satisfied. Few of her problems had such simple solutions.

For four years I indulged in silent reading almost exclusively. There were some arithmetic classes, some essays, two or three carved trays, and a compulsory share of community singing. Then I would retreat into my private world. There were a few volumes by E. S. Ellis, Capt. Marryatt, R. G. Ballantyne and G. H. Henty. These, pure stuff for boys, were soon exhausted and I had to move on to sterner works. I read *The Last of the Mohicans, John Halifax Gentleman, Westward Ho!, The Swiss Family Robinson, Lorna Doone, Robinson Crusoe, Treasure Island, Don Quixote* (the last I thought incredibly silly). Large portions were obscure but I, lacking all guidance, had to experiment. I was an early convert to Dickens through *Pickwick Papers*, when I sometimes startled the school by laughing out loud at the aphorisms of Sam Weller. The selection began to shrink and I read Scott, Thackeray and George Eliot, but most of this was beyond my comprehension. I read mainly for the story. I always wanted to know what happened to the characters. I never considered what might be happening to me. As an introduction to general education it was disastrous. As an introduction to the specialty of English it was magnificent. They were impressionable years. There was ample storage in the memory for a large vocabulary and imperceptibly there developed a discrimination in phrasing, a sensitivity to meaning, a confidence in the use of well-chosen words and an appreciative recognition of a shapely sentence. As the vocabulary increased, the easier recall of the appropriate words lent fluency to speech, where, once the idea was shaped the words selected themselves.

When I reached school leaving age I had to put the books away. I sat – unsuccessfully – an Education Board Scholarship, going in to Timaru each day for the purpose. It was my first examination. I did not complete any paper. In 'General Science' I answered the easy domestic questions and was informed later that they were the alternatives meant for the girls. One paper was 'English'. I did not know what it meant and had spent the previous evening poring over a map of the British Isles.

In retrospect the one who came out of it best was Miss Johnston, tirelessly and with dignity doing her best at an impossible task. This is a country slow to acknowledge that teachers, the selected dedicated ones, if given small classes and full facilities can hold in their hands the key to the future. The legislators are endlessly concerned with strictures on the malefactors without seeming to realize that every malefactor is an educational casualty. Youth is always looking for a place to hang its enthusiasm. A good teacher always has suggestions. The community life of Fairview such as it was depended largely on Miss Johnston. She was secretary of the Mutual Improvement Society, postmistress day or night if someone wanted to make a telephone call. Morning telegrams she had to deliver by any method she could devise. She had a class of music pupils. Until my father relieved her she held a Sunday School. At the school house was her invalid mother. There was also a horse and trap and a vegetable garden to maintain.

For all this she received one hundred and sixty five pounds a year.

I left school at the traditional age of thirteen with a Sixth Standard Proficiency certificate. I have no idea how I got this but it was real, for I remember a serving-maid handling it enviously and saying, 'You don't know how lucky you are'.

For most, thirteen marked the end of the educational adventure. At that age they could nearly all read and write, could hold up their end in a financial transaction and could make an occasional reckless contribution to an argument. After that it was hobnailed boots for the boys and long pinafores for the girls and on the farm the old cycle would start again. There were two functions every year which convinced the parents that schooling and education were synonymous. One was the winter social and dance in aid of the prize-giving fund. The admission was two and six, ladies a plate, and the expenses were nil. The profits were therefore twenty to thirty pounds, and this was invested in prize books of which the most costly was five shillings and the average two and sixpence.

At the end of the year came the annual prize-giving and break-up. The same local artists contributed the usual concert after which came the prize-giving by the chairman of the school committee. His table was piled high with shiny new books. They were handed to him in turn by Miss Johnston, almost unrecognizable in a long black frock. There then ensued the extraordinary dissipation of prizes. Every pupil received a minimum of three to four prizes for excellence in an imaginative range of subjects. There were prizes for general ability, for most improvement during the year, for pre-eminence in any one Standard. Also there were three prizes at least for the three top places in each subject in each Standard. The school committee insisted that the funds having been collected for prizes should be spent on prizes and Miss Johnston deserves credit for the imaginative way in which she got rid of them all. It involved occasionally giving a pupil first prize in a subject of which he had never heard. The worst feature of it was that we saw nothing incongruous in it. We marched up, insufferably egoistic, and received our prizes as of right with no scruples

46

about any prerequisite of merit. Later, in the upper sixth at the high school, familiarity with irregular Latin verbs or the nuances of Horace's odes might be rewarded by one volume of the classics. Such volumes I still possess and treasure. The loot from Fairview has gone and only my grandchildren know where.

My brother and I, having minimal problems of reading, were almost unassailable in the matter of prizes. Again and again we would march up and return with a volume that we would park beneath my mother's wheelchair. One year, so heavy were our acquisitions that we carried them up the road and stacked them inside our gate. My brother then went home for the wheelbarrow.

Fairview approved. The dullest child was, competitively, better than some other child. There resulted a gratifying equality of superiority. Every family had its triumphant member. The prize-giving was proof of a year of indefatigable industry. Now – on with the dance.

The booksellers, P. W. Hutton & Co. of Timaru, usually gave a special prize as discount. One year this was for the most popular boy in the school to be decided by vote, two votes for first choice and one for second. The girls nominated a sleek young Lothario and the boys a bullet-headed young thug. It became obvious that the second vote was tricky. It should not be given to a rival, it should be thrown away on a nonentity. Somehow I was nominated for this position. I accordingly got one vote from almost everyone in the school, two votes from myself (almost certainly) and two each from my brothers if they kept their promises. I liked to think also, that I had one or two secret admirers among the girls. The result was that I topped the poll and when, in relative silence, I went up to get my prize as the most popular boy, I could sense the intense hostility of the whole school. It was a sharp lesson in one of the fallacies of democracy. But it was a good prize: *Deeds that Won the Empire*. Never for a moment did I consider the propriety of giving it back.

I too was to be a farmer, but first I had to have a secondary education, and to this I happily agreed as did two of my brothers in their turn. It was an unorthodox approach to agriculture and inevitably incurred criticism. 'Trying to make his sons better than their father, is he?'

I left Fairview School gladly because of the greater adventures ahead. I have been back of course, most recently within a year, but there is now no magnet. The new school, the staff of two, the formed roads, mown lawns, the gardens, the rare trees all appropriately labelled, the memorial gates, the bike stand – all these have replaced the memory pegs of the past. Only the site is common to the two eras. I was welcomed by the headmaster and we tried doggedly to establish a common interest in his future and my past. I explained how my personality and in fact my whole life had been modified by four years of silent reading in his school. He seemed puzzled. Apparently it would no longer be possible. A pity.

The Timaru Boys' High School in 1912 backed on to the Girls' School and there were many who thought the proximity unseemly especially for the dangerous unsegregated common pathway of about a chain before the girls veered off behind the enormous hedge. In the interests of propriety the two schools were assembled and dismissed at different times. During my first month there was a scandal. A boy and girl, engaged in vigorous conversation biked through the gate and occupied the whole of their common route with discussion. The scandal wilted a little when it was revealed that the culprits were brother and sister continuing a breakfast table argument.

The first day at secondary school was intimidating. I had to make my own way there and I was uncertain even as to its location. Rumour had it that a gruelling examination was to determine our placings in the third form. We went in awe of the town scholars. They were sophisticated men-about-town, knowledgeable on all matters including the limitations of their country cousins. But instead of the exam there was an essay, 'A Day in the Life of a Dog'. I lost all my apprehension as I became immersed in this. Our old sheep-dog, Mack, and I had been buddies for years. I projected myself into his personality, wrote in the first person and emphasized human foibles and canine superiority. That night I was troubled. My imaginative fling would have earned a tick from Miss Johnston but would probably be regarded as flippant in the more austere circles of secondary education. I never received any criticism of the essay, but the next day I was promoted to the fourth form for English, the only new kid to receive this distinction. This was the first slow leak in the town-country bubble. (Complete deflation was achieved five years later when of the six members of the University Scholarship class in the upper sixth, four were the sons of small farmers.)

I remember little of that year. I suppose there was some form of organized sport followed by the annual sports day but I have no recollection of them, nor of the Waitaki match. I have no recollection of the break-up ceremony, yet there must have been one for I was presented with a prize for Botany, the only science prize I have ever won in my life. My school day began with a breathless rush to be on time and finished with the dismissal bell when I turned my bike to the limpid sky above the Alps, the sting and blast of the nor'-westers and at home a welcoming mooing from the cows in the yard dragging their too heavy udders.

The only subject I remember in that year was English. Our master was

Mr Rockel. He was a broad, heavy, slowfooted Teutonic gentleman and presumably because of schoolboy fondness for antithesis was known as 'Fairy'. But he loved English poetry and he easily taught me to love it too. There was no more silent reading. He went over every poem with us, line by line, often word by word. By this method we 'did' during that year 'Lycidas', *Julius Caesar*, *The Merchant of Venice*, 'The Ancient Mariner', 'La Belle Dame' and 'John Gilpin' as well as shorter lyrics. We had to memorize large sections. I found these easy to learn and a pleasure to master, and at all times a stimulus to public speaking. Out in a back paddock I would stand on a hillside and with dramatic gestures deliver Mark Antony's oration to the mildly surprised sheep. At the end of that year Mr Rockel left for New Plymouth Boys' High School. Later I knew his son who died, as a first-year medical student, of pernicious anaemia.

It was not a proud school in those days. The Headmaster, Mr Simmers, was a noted mathematician, but this was not enough. There was a boarding establishment with three residents only. The only football ground was on the curve of a hill so steep that fifteen boy scouts could have held the All Blacks at bay till half-time provided they won the toss. In later years under the white-hot enthusiasm of Mr Thomas, the journey to and from Waitaki had all the colour of the launching of an Armada.

The next year we vacated in favour of the girls and reassembled at the brand new school in North Street where even the staff (with the one exception of Mr Munro) was new. We of the fourth form swaggered about as if we had been the architects and were insufferable to the new cringing third formers (who included my brother). Our new Rector, Mr W. Thomas, had been headmaster of the Waimataitai primary school. We thought little of this as a credential. It was rather like putting in the first eleven someone who was good at French cricket. We built up a picture of him which he shattered on the first day when he divided the whole school into elevens and ran a series of cricket matches. The next day he gave the first of his famous talks, a clarion-call to action and we who came to sneer remained to cheer. That year he promised that we would form an orchestra and a band and fill the Timaru theatre for two nights with a public concert. (There was no organized music of any sort in the school.) We would beat Waitaki at football (we had not scored against them for twelve years) and the school would get three University Scholarships (we had never heard of them). All these prophecies were fulfilled. The scholarship winners were (I think) Scott, Stevens and Valentine.

In recent years Mr Thomas has been the subject of a biographical sketch by a later contemporary master. Inevitably, it misses his psychological approach to the young male. He believed that the school was full of mute inglorious Miltons and that it was the duty of the school to uncover the talent. The routine syllabus was not enough. There was formal instruction in art, drama, chess, astronomy, oratory, debating, photography, gymnastics, music, singing, athletics. He knew that in every boy is the zeal to excel, the hunger to be pre-eminent in some small field. No deed of distinction by any scholar would pass unnoticed by him. Thus we strove, fiercely, competitively, to the limit of our ability and our ability was the greater thereby.

But that was in another day. Some modern educationalists deplore scholastic competition. It perverts the winner and depresses the loser. It has no place in the general education which is the purpose of schooling. So the pedestals have been removed; the standard forms have been trundled out. The University Scholarship winners must not be identified by their school or contrasted by their marks. Fame is the spur, but it is no plant that grows on common soil. Why not comparable reticence about military decorations, athletic records, Birthday Honours?

Mr Thomas's methods were well illustrated at his first Waitaki match. That morning at the assembly of the whole school he won the match on his own. He named every man in the team and one by one, convinced him that all the glory, prestige and honour of the Timaru Boys' High School was in his keeping that afternoon. The team believed it and so did the rest of the school. As a result there marched onto the field fifteen inspired little Timaru demons. The next morning at assembly he rose to speak in an expectant silence. 'Well,' he said casually, 'We won.' There was an outburst of applause. When it quietened he began to analyse, not the match, but the players. He started with the captain and concluded his eulogy with: 'And surely he was a hero'. Then he referred briefly to fourteen others and in every instance finished with: 'And he was a hero too'. It was spine-tingling stuff. The catalyst of loyalty between pupil and school was often sport. Mr E. A. Cockroft, one of the masters, was an All Black. Mr Thomas himself was a South Canterbury cricket representative. When a visiting Australian team compiled an astronomical score against South Canterbury, and one of their leading batsmen (was it Trumper?) threatened to preserve the last wicket indefinitely, Mr Thomas was brought on to bowl. His first ball scattered the wickets and closed the innings. As a result he was given the favour of opening the next innings with Trumper bowling. The ball came down and was slammed for six. The loyalty of the school to its head was thereby cemented for years.

The morning assembly set the school pulsating for the day. Here was the news: school, local, international. Praise, censure, operation orders, demands, were all paraded at the morning assembly. On the board was a gigantic map of France and whenever there was activity on the Western Front he moved the little red flags back and forth. After the assembly the school slipped into a rigid routine of forty-five minute teaching periods covering the subjects of English, Latin, French, Mathematics, Agriculture and either Drawing or History. At the end of the third year Matriculation demanded a five subject pass, though the school expected all its candidates to pass in six. He did not believe that education had to be contained within the examination system. The committee of enquiry into secondary education of which he was chairman issued its famous 'Thomas Report' in 1944 and advocated a more liberal range of subjects, School Certificate and accrediting.

The school was far more than a system of classes. Sport was organized – football, cricket, fives, swimming, athletics and gymnastics – and hotly contested. My participation in all this was comprehensive, maximal, enthusiastic and generally mediocre. After school the extra-curricular subjects flourished. Every boy had his liberty but it was not a secret liberty.

The first six years in the new school were times of war either pending or waging and in many ways the school was affected. In 1912 came compulsory cadet training. For me this meant that every Wednesday I climbed into a pair of khaki shorts (issue) so large that both my legs would have gone into one half. I then biked to school with a .303 rifle on my back. After school we paraded, answered the roll, marched round the football field and were dismissed. Under the stimulus of war our military 'training' expanded. We learned a set of parade-ground manoeuvres which were no longer operative during the second war. I became a sergeant. No one was impressed. It was all a gross waste of effort. In fact military training has never been distinguished by efficiency. Once a year we had to do a long route march. The route, the pace and the destination mattered not. All that counted was that we had to do it in uniform and for a minimum period of time. Again once a year down on the shingled shore of Timaru we shot off a few rounds, and the kick of a .303 against the shoulder of a young boy is more conducive to pacifism than to good marksmanship. We once held a 'battle'. The school was divided into two halves and allotted opposing bush-clad hillsides. We then infiltrated enemy territory until we had fired off our ration of blanks. The whole training of five years was inferior to what a crusty staff sergeant at Trentham could have taught in two days.

But at the time we made little protest. We were at the age when an egoistic strut is almost inevitable and there was much satisfaction in exhibiting rifle and uniform on the road home. As far as I knew I was the only legally appointed defender of Fairview. I hoped the locals were impressed, for no one at home was. 'Take that gun out of here,' ordered my mother who had a gay abandon with synonyms. After all she used to call my brother's tennis racquet a 'bat'.

One afternoon when I was changing out of football boots in the locker room there came from outside an excited shouting. Wearing one shoe and one football boot I went out. 'New Zealanders in action! Pushing the enemy back. Hooray, hooray, now it won't be long.' We cheered them and, God forgive us, we envied them. We went looking for the Dardenelles first on the map of France. Some of those who cheered that day were to die in France in the next few years. One of the most popular young masters at the time was Dan O'Connor, whose brother Mick was a pupil, and later, in the war shortage, became a pupil teacher for a year and then enlisted. Both were killed in action.

Naturally the war depleted the staff which ceased to be selective. Mr Thomas taught senior English but he lacked the inherent enthusiasm of Mr Rockel. Perhaps the best teacher was Mr Tait with the rare gift of being able to impart mathematical knowledge. Mr Ongley and his successor Miss Duthie (later Lady Barrowclough) were better classical scholars than classical teachers. Three pupil teachers were appointed from the sixth form. No science was taught except Agriculture which was a bait for farmers' sons. It stopped at Matriculation, which could easily be passed if one had an essay in mind on the rotation of crops, knew the formula for Bordeaux Mixture and the mechanism of the Babcock milktester. For those requiring a science for University Scholarship the choice fell on Chemistry for which the school provided a chemistry laboratory, recommended two text books, (Newth's *Chemistry* in two volumes) and assured us that the subject was a real challenge to us in that we had to master it without a teacher. At Chemistry periods we would repair to the laboratory and doggedly try again to read the subject. But the reading confused and did not teach. Occasionally Mr O'Connor, nominally in charge of the Chemistry class, would look in the door and say 'What's $H_2SO_4 + NaCl$?' In chorus we would shout the answer. 'Good,' he would say, 'carry on.' It was his only equation and almost our only one. We would then go back to the sports of phosphorus on water or mercury globules on a bench. Inevitably our attempt at the University Scholarship paper in Chemistry was pure farce. If I had been allowed to set the paper myself I am sure I could not have passed. The night before the examination I selected a page from Volume One and another one from Volume Two. I then learned them off by heart having no idea of the meaning. The next morning I answered each of the first four questions by half a page of the memorized text. What I wrote was of course perfect – a textbook cannot be wrong – but I doubt if there was any association between the question and the answer for I could not understand either. For this, in due course I was awarded six per cent. I think this must have been for audacity. But I could never understand how the dux of the school (Martin Fowler) got three per cent. Perhaps he memorized only one page. Small as the marks were, the consequences were smaller for no marks under twenty-five per cent were counted in the final. This was a university edict for reasons quite obscure, unless they were Biblical. 'For unto every one that hath shall be given, and he shall have abundance: but from him that hath not shall be taken away even that which he hath.' Matthew 25: 29.

Then came the day of my last break-up. My locker had been cleared, my text books removed. I had received my special prefect's memento from Mr Thomas. For the last time I listened to someone advising the leavers on the formula for success in life. I had no need of such instruction. I had had five years at one of the best schools in the country, had worked hard and was fully equipped for life. I had taken prizes in essays, languages and debating. I probably knew more Swinburne than anyone in the school. I had gone confidently with Caesar through Gaul. But I had not been further north than Christchurch, nor further south than Oamaru. I could not have drawn a map of New Zealand, nor have put in any historical setting Wakefield, Vogel, Grey, Godley or Ballance. I could not have understood a balance sheet (I still have trouble) or the difference between stocks and shares, the conduct of parliament, the ingredients of politics. I fully subscribed to all the chivalry of the Arthurian knights but when faced with a member of the other sex I was as graceful as a cow in a quadrille.

What to do? I could be a competent farmer but my father, now crippled with arthritis, favoured a profession and so did I. My secret ambition was to be a poet – with a few prose masterpieces thrown in. This could best be achieved by becoming a teacher with sufficient leisure to allow the full maturing of genius. When in doubt teach. I was in doubt more than I knew, so teaching it had to be. Parental approval was automatic. Yet, a few days later:

'Wouldn't it be lovely to become a doctor?' suggested my mother, looking at her twisted fingers.

'I would like to put you through the medical course,' said my father. 'But I'm afraid it's too expensive.'

I applied therefore for a position as pupil teacher at the Christchurch West school, was appointed, packed my bag and said goodbye. For the first (and last) time in my life I missed the train. I sent a wire cancelling my appointment and then, after a dilatory period of wavering indecision and repetitive discussion, I caught the train for Dunedin, became domiciled at Knox College and enrolled as a medical student which involved presenting a Matriculation certificate, paying a fee and filling up a form. Of all the students enrolled that year I was undoubtedly the least suitable. I knew nothing of medicine. My motives were humanitarian but were sicklied o'er with sentiment. I wanted to solve the mystery of my mother's illness and after that restore health and happiness to anyone in affliction. The medical course is involved all through with the sciences in two of which most students had been grounded at school. The only science I knew concerned the predictable behaviour of H_2SO_4 under certain defined conditions. At the present day I certainly would not have been accepted as a medical student. But the modern insistence on high entry marks in the sciences is all wrong. Medicine is an art. It deals with human beings and not with the shaped bricks of science. The poor student who becomes an excellent doctor is a commonplace in the medical history of New Zealand.

The miserable year that followed must, in pity, be lightly sketched. I arrived late and the first precious days of orientation were over. I went to lectures in Physics and found that it had nothing to do with the physic of pharmacology. The lecturer, Professor Jack, was a Scot of enormous energy and enthusiasm and with an accent which was like icicles breaking under cartwheels. Not only could I not understand what he was teaching but I could not even understand what he was saying. Other students were working with an energy which perturbed me.

Surely medicine did not require such effort? I sprained my ankle and was absent for nearly a fortnight. There was ominous talk of the Medical Intermediate in six months and the necessity to keep terms. I made weighty new resolutions, opened the text books again at the first chapter, wrote some lyrics and then had my appendix removed. Everyone was very helpful. Other students offered to lend me their notes. Professors Jack and Inglis kindly allowed me to do my arrears of practical work after hours. Professor Benham refused a similar privilege (being short of frogs and rabbits for dissection). This meant that I could not keep terms in this subject. I floundered on with a maximum strain on memory and a minimum on comprehension. Yet I kept terms in Physics and Chemistry and passed Intermediate in the latter.

There was a term still to go and those who passed went on to the excitement of Anatomy and Dissection. I tried to join them on an amateur basis so to speak. I was not allowed and for this I was glad. The dissecting room with its orderly rows of metal topped tables incongruously associated with death, dismemberment and carbolic, was repellent. I knew this was not squeamishness but I did not know it was immaturity. I went home. My parents said little. They were sad and puzzled. So was I. It was not the right time to tell them that I had finished with medicine. Next year I would be a pupil teacher in Christchurch. Or would be something or other somewhere. Better anything than being adrift at nineteen. I was beginning to lose faith in silent reading and La Fontaine and iambic pentameters. The world was more jagged than I had imagined. Preparation for it involved rougher training by rougher teachers. Meanwhile I got into old clothes, took the milk bucket out of my father's hand and went back to the cows.

4

The Fabric of a Farm

At first sight it was a splendid farm, over three hundred acres in a more or less rectangular block with good gates, strong fences of gorse growing on a clay wall, plenty of outbuildings and a cobbled cowyard. The house, viewed from the main road nearly half a mile away had dignity and charm, large, single-storeyed, cream painted, with a lawn and a garden and extensive plantations.

On second sight the property had some similarity to a very good second-hand car newly-painted. The previous owner had inherited a legacy and spent it on trying to change a farmhouse into a gentleman's residence. He built a broad verandah round two sides and small bedrooms on the other two sides, one of which opened from the kitchen, another from the drawing room, two from the verandah and one from outside. The bathroom was in the centre and the approach could never be described except by diagrams. In all there were at least seven bedrooms. Though an architectural nightmare, it suited us by providing a bedroom each.

The farm was composed of 'rolling downs', which meant that the gullies could be artificially blocked to form drains for watering stock. It also meant that the water-race which supplied Timaru with water and which meandered about in pursuit of levels destroyed any symmetry in the paddocks. The race ran between two heavy wire fences about a chain apart. The gullies themselves were bridged by three flumes, massive conduits about two feet wide, latticed across the top with steel braces and supported on metal pylons rising out of the gully. We frequently walked across the flumes, balancing precariously and dangerously on the steel braces.

By our time the open race had been flowing since 1881 through farmlands from the Pareora River over twenty miles away. Despite having permanent maintenance men every few miles it was far from a perfect system. Not infrequently the water-race men would shovel out dead birds and the smaller animals. It was replaced in 1939 by a sixteen inch pipe which was more efficient but less interesting. The dams ceased to be dams when they could no longer be filled by anchoring in the flume a branch covered by a sack. The goldfish, frogs and chicks disappeared. The downlands water supply became available in 1941 with ample water for households and farms. Till then all farmers had to rely on roof supply. Our own water storage system was elaborate. The water drained through filters just below the spouting and into two underground concrete tanks which in effect formed the backyard of the house. We had been informed that the tanks had a capacity of fifteen thousand gallons each and this we proudly repeated without any proof of its accuracy. From these tanks the water was pumped to a supply tank by a windmill. As a result we always had ample high pressure water. We believed in our water system and left it to look after itself. But it would have been better if the birds had left the roof alone, and the spoutings had not been blocked with rotting leaves and pine needles, and the wire gauze in the filters had persisted intact, and there had been no surface drainage through the cracks in the concrete tanks, and if the water itself had, somehow, acquired a little fluorine. Yet we seemed to suffer no ill effects other than dental.

It was a mixed farm which meant that in addition to the three main ventures of cows, sheep and grain, there was a crowded background of supportive affairs all essential to successful farming: feed (hay, swedes and mangolds); repair of gates and fences; gorse grubbing; raising, feeding and slaughtering pigs; maintaining a vegetable garden; periodic sale of hams; preserving of eggs; sun drying of apples; bottling fruit; topping pine trees; feeding animals; repairing machinery, horse-collars, and sacks; tarpainting the outbuildings; clearing out the cowyard and stacking the winter firewood. 'Finished for the night,' my mother would say. 'Yes, finished – for the night.'

No mixed farm has the right soil for all purposes. Ours was a poor soil, too full of clay and too starved of humus. It was mainly steep slopes and the winter rains gouged deep channels. It was also heavily riddled with twitch. Our method of dealing with this was to skim-plough in the autumn and when the furrow was dry shake the soil loose with a pitch fork, pile the tangle of roots in little mounds and burn it. It was a method utterly ineffective. The remaining roots were stimulated to greater vigour in the following year.

It was a soil quite unsuitable for the continuous cropping of wheat. Wheat is a hungry substance. It leaves little in the soil and demands rotation at longer periods than a small farm can afford. Yet for most of his farming days my father patriotically persisted with wheat. The country needed it, said the Government urgently during the war. Furthermore the smooth cycle of growing wheat had a special charm. It began with the autumn ploughing and sowing, each drill box receiving its standard quantity of superphosphate. Thereafter the farmer could do little (except to keep swarms of small birds on the move) until the harvest. By harvest time the crop could be appraised. It might be ragged and stunted owing to the drought, or lying down beyond redemption because of a week-long drizzle, or (especially oats) so infested with rust that after two rounds of the binder the driver was the same colour as the horses. But it could also be a fine undulating yellow canopy, fence high, capable of fifty bushels an acre. Wheat growing is not entirely free from the gambler's lure.

There were two kinds. Velvet, a strong grower, was gentle to handle but notorious for shedding the grain. So that if some grain had lost its milkiness and a nor'-west wind began to drift down from the hills, the binder had to be raced out and arrangements made for relays of horses and men driving through the night. The other was solid straw Tuscan, heavy, a good flour producer, full of spikes and barbs and brutal to handle. Stacking was best done by a gang of five and was usually on a co-operative basis with neighbouring farmers. It could also be done awkwardly by three using one dray and this is the method we often adopted. From starting as a lowly crow I later became a competent stacker. When the threshing machine came it had a complete autonomy. The farmer stood off, counting the sacks of grain and assessing his year's return and had no other responsibility than to keep up the supply of empty sacks for if these failed the standard charge of thirty five shillings an hour continued.

The final stage was the marketing. Usually my father and I would go to town, I driving the trap while he pored over the samples he was to submit, picking out and discarding all the imperfect grains. This was standard practice acknowledged as such by vendor and purchaser. The sale was to an agency, usually the one that held the mortgage on the farm. There was no guaranteed price, no competition to firm up the market. The farmer might demur but in the end he took what he was offered. It was never as much as he hoped. The cheque would be lodged against his overdraft. He would thus be guaranteed another frugal year and would go back home and start ploughing for the autumn sowings.

As on all mixed farms there were those foolproof investments the cows. Except in winter they looked after themselves, often in awkward corners and were usually milked by women and children, or, in our yard, by my brother and myself. Always there were two cows in milk and in the season as many as twelve. In the five years I went to the High School I estimate that I sat down to milk a cow over eighteen hundred times. There was occasional help from my father. Then my brother won a boarding scholarship and appeared in the yard only at week-ends.

Even now my prejudices against cows have not mellowed. The cow is the stupidest of animals. It chews the cud with banal placidity while making up its mind for the sole purpose of changing it. The two exceptions to this vacillation are when it discovers a hole in the fence round the vegetable garden or when in the bail it discovers the leg rope has been overlooked.

Before we invested in a separator the milk was placed in shallow pans and skimmed twice in forty-eight hours. The cream went into earthenware jars and the milk went to the pigs or calves, the latter enjoying as well a little fresh milk. Once a week we made butter. It was a straight sequence: churn to butter, run off the buttermilk, work the milk out with buttercloth, work the salt in, weigh, pat up into pounds, wrap and store for sale. It was usually horrible butter, deeply yellow, rank and tainted. It was sold to the grocer who had no option but to accept it if he wished the trade to be reciprocal. We often produced fifty pounds of butter a week.

I never came to terms with the cows. I would arrive home from school, look at the paper, noting the bits my mother had cut out so that I could find in the library the next day the minor reports of casting offensive matter, exposure while drunk, and putative fathership. Then would come a meal, a change into greasy old milking clothes and I would take my buckets and depart to the stupid creatures round the yard gate. At about the same time my scholastic rivals at the Rectory would be congregating for their formal prep.

The sheep were homely adjuncts to a farm, asking little and yielding much. Their care was restricted to the short episodes of shearing, crutching, dipping, docking, spaying and supervision in the lambing season. In return were sales of lambs and wool and skins, and year-round mutton on the table. Behind the cowyard was a small piece of rich pasture in which there were a dozen or more choice sheep. It was a veritable death row. My father would stride into the huddle of sheep in the corner and drag out one by the hind leg. Twenty minutes later it had been butchered and the joints were hanging in the gauzed meatsafe under the fir tree. We used mutton extravagantly at a time when no other extravagance was permitted. This was because we could not kill half a sheep at a time. A full sheep without refrigeration was too much for one family and often the last leg had to be boiled and served with a strong caper sauce. Cats and dogs had plenty and occasionally the pigs shared. Certain relatives in Timaru always appreciated a joint. It was our main source of meat. Rabbits and hares came next, then, rarely, pork and, more rarely still, a fowl. Occasionally four farmers would club together and acquire a quarter of beef each.

The sheep, being prime, filled many kerosene tins with fat and this had numerous uses. Some of it was sold and some made into soap. It was the universal lubricant and also (unsalted) the remedy for all cuts, abrasions and skin lesions. In winter the fat-laden peritoneum of a killed sheep was usually festooned over nails on the wall of a shed and was soon covered by swarms of wax-eyes and fantails.

Sheep seem to live in a world which they completely fail to understand. They will follow a leader grateful that the leader has done the thinking for them. While my father or I have been killing a sheep, they have given us a little uncomprehending attention and have then resumed grazing. They are needlessly frightened of all dogs, a weakness which the dogs shamelessly exploit. Once, on my way to the Woodbury school, there came from behind me a runaway mob, crowding fence to fence and preventing the drover or the dogs from herding them. I, about the size of one of them, dashed from side to side, yelling and flapping arms. They stopped in complete bewilderment. The drover pushed through and so did his outraged dogs. The man gave me threepence which was the first money I ever earned. The sheep population of the country was recorded in the Appendices to the Journal of the House. In 1908, our first year at Fairview, we had two hundred and twenty one and, three years later, four hundred and eighteen.

For many years we had a ploughman who, if single, lived in the house or if married occupied the other house on the farm with a few acres of land. The standard wage was one pound a week with keep. Also there was a succession of maids ranging from the estimable down to the worthless. As I look back on it one's sympathy has to be with the maid. She was housekeeper to the family, nurse to my mother, foster mother to some strong-willed boys, a twelve-hour-a-day slave. The wages varied but were almost certain to be less than that of the ploughman. But she was freely admitted into the family and given a good home. This, after all, was her objective. They were austere times for a single girl. If she had no qualifications for teaching or for being a governess, there was the narrow choice of work in a hotel, a factory or a home. Only in the last could there be a reasonable chance of benevolent friendship. Two of our maids, even after they left, remained friends of the family for years.

Among our more colourful neighbours was Willie Long and his gang of Chinese market gardeners. They lived on our side of a hill in a shanty town of packing cases and corrugated iron and they rented five acres across the road from my father. At dawn there were always several of them at work and several more as the sun set, giving the impression that they had been working all night. Their only holiday seemed to be their traditional New

Year when they awoke the district with crackers and fireworks and devoted the day to feasting. My father was always a guest on these occasions and would come home laden with Chinese sweetmeats, usually dry, tangy and sweet. He was loud in his praise of his tenants and of their national brandy. Despite their addiction to their somewhat tasteless preserves they usually bought one or more of our sucking pigs before the festival.

Our own vegetable-growing was based on what one man, one horse and one cultivator could do in one day of the year on the rich loamy patch at the side of the house. By mid-afternoon it would be striated with ridges and the sowing would begin. As many packets had lost their labels and some twists of seeds had never had a label and friends and neighbours had left samples of something now forgotten and as the sower could never remember where he had sown what, the result was full of interest and sometimes of excitement. After the sowing there was a perfunctory thinning and then no more till the maid went looking for a supplement to the day's meals. We seemed to have no caterpillars or aphides.

When our vegetable supply ran low someone, usually myself, would be sent down to Willie Long with an empty sugar bag. While he filled the bag he would emphasize the hard times, the high cost of vegetable growing and his impending bankruptcy. I would refute all this and substitute the lamentable state of the small farmer. We argued not to convince but to amuse. Eventually he would shove the bag at me, extend his hand and say 'a shilling', at which I would recoil in horror and offer threepence. Then the haggle began and it carefully followed an old script. The final compromise was usually for sixpence which now seems so unrealistic that I suspect he and my father had some secret arrangement. Finally, in the best of good humour we parted, each going down his own special path to bankruptcy.

In those days all farming was risky. There was no government help in times of disaster, no guaranteed price, no scientific help that was available in practicable form. The farmer had to make his own decisions, act on them and be his own salesman. Despite his best efforts he could be ruined and everyone would agree that it was bad luck, but like death itself, had to be accepted. He always worked even in prosperous days with a sense of having his back to the wall. There resulted a bitter harvest of parsimony. Nothing was ever bought that was not a full necessity, and the house and farm became a workshop for improvisations. Our mother made our clothes, patching, repatching and handing on. Under her direction I made a shirt for myself at the age of twelve which was a creditable achievement and a manufacturing disaster. My first bought suit (three pounds ten shillings) was a blue serge, when I was thirteen. We repaired our own shoes, made preserving bottles by cutting off any conical necks, used paper spills instead of matches, manufactured our own soap. Regularly our father would line us all up for haircuts. On the farm were tarpaulin substitutes of sacks sewn together, the saddlery bound with twine, tangles of wire in the gaps of the fences, 'Taranaki' gates and deep fords filled with pine branches. In the corners of sheds, behind doors, under the hedges were the rope, wire, axles, discarded machinery all waiting vainly for a possible use. It was therefore an untidy farm. So was every farm in the vicinity for each put up the same feeble defence against recoil of the mortgage. Every show farm of today has had to pay for it. Fifty years ago no farmer would dare divert any assets for development as long as he still had a mortgage.

As a result the farmer was not mentally conditioned to progress. My father followed the same old sequence as his father had done Given the luck of a good season it promised a safer margin of security than any risky new enterprise. On a number of occasions he went to Lincoln College on Farmers' Day. He was back by evening and for days would tell of the marvellous advances he had seen. But he never considered adopting any of them even in humble modified form, for they would have to have had a foundation of money.

There was of course no leisure on the farm. Our only relaxation was either defined by school activities or was based on our extraordinary involvement with reading. Always we had our quota of standard duties, but if ever free time supervened there was a moral obligation to hack down thistles, fat hen and docks, to cut gorse fences, grub gorse on the hillsides, thin swede turnips, top pines, chop firewood. Round this our personalities were shaped. We became natural and tireless toilers, resistant to all the claims of relaxation or amusement. It was far from a desirable state. Yet no one misses what he has not had and our boyhood was to us eminently satisfactory. In the winter evenings when the farm was shut away, the green plush cover with the long tassels would be thrown over the kitchen table and the kerosene lamp placed in the centre. Then the family would be in quiet intimacy, my father deep in the *Timaru Herald* or the *Farmers' Journal*, my mother, sight permitting, finishing her day with one of her two favourite authors, St Paul or Charles Dickens. On the other side of the lamp would be my brother and myself grunting over the elusive figure represented by *x* or tossing with Aeneas in the Mediterranean. My youngest two brothers would be in bed (or at least had been sent there).

All through our school days my brother and I never lost our obsession with reading. We displayed much ingenuity in obtaining reading material and then, though apparently otherwise engaged, in appropriating time to read it. Our library was spread under our pillows, in strawstacks, under hedges, in the box of the dray. We had wire frames for books attached to the wall by the separator, on the handles of our bikes. I had an ingenious tripod by my milking stool, but my brother used a wire frame drooped over the back of the indignant cow. When we were assigned to 'going round the sheep' we would scamper on to one or two vantage points, gaze carefully from fence to fence and then read for half an hour before reporting that the sheep were all right. One day my brother and I were ploughing a long narrow paddock. We were accompanied by our old sheepdog Mack, a creature of extraordinary intelligence. Mack was, in fact, one of our sturdiest employees. He slept on the verandah, and my father at six a.m. would call 'Mack' and Mack would acknowledge the order with two thumps of his tail and go off and bring the cows into the yard. On the ploughing occasion Mack did the ploughing. The team would arrive at one end, Mack with a firm hold on the reins. One of the two ploughmen would turn the plough and the team round, hand the reins to Mack and go back to a book.

While at primary school we had access to the *Boys Own Paper*, usually in three-monthly volumes. They were, I think, borrowed from some source. This was a grand little periodical but it was insignificant beside its robust rival *Chums*. There was everything in *Chums*: suspense, terror, courage that was never less than foolhardy, incredible coincidences and the universal triumph of right – or might, which often meant the same thing. There were times when the reader could barely endure the predicament of the hero (who was nearly always a male of the late teens). Most days finished with ten precious minutes of *Chums* read in bed with a candle on the pillow (all strictly forbidden). In *Chums* were Cowboys and Indians, pirates, mysteries of the Sargasso sea and countless near-perils of the Empire. One serial had as its hero the fifth former who was the sole relative of an elderly millionaire uncle. The nephew was to be his heir provided he was prepared to spend the fortune and not hoard it. The boy's capacity to do this was put to the trial by giving him five thousand pounds to get rid of in one term. There were all sorts of tags: no gifts, no dissipation, no purchases except for personal use. Week by week we followed breathlessly the futile efforts of the spender. Everything he touched turned to gold. Halfway through the term his original capital had doubled. I suppose he won through in the end. They always did. Later, my admiration for his ingenuity was exceeded by admiration for the author's cheek in formulating a plot so banal.

Chums came to us through favour of some cousins, the Faber-Browns who lived at Te Moana. As they finished with each copy their mother would post it to us. One day my father picked up a copy and read a short story where the baddie was made to walk the plank and then was pelted with broken bottles until he sank beneath the multitudinous seas incarnadine. My father, greatly displeased with his sister, went off to my mother who was horrified. In vain we pleaded that it was an exceptional story. My mother wrote to my aunt expressing thanks for the past and a firm embargo on the future. Poor mother. She believed in Original Sin but believed without reason that her boys had escaped. It was my duty to post the letters and collect the mail. She never asked me whether the letter had been posted. Thereafter *Chums* had to be kept out of sight, under the mattress or in the bottom of a drawer, where my father wouldn't look and my mother couldn't look and a maid could look and be none the wiser.

Steadily the range of literature widened. At the High School, poetry lit up a new world of imagination, beauty and colour. It was no world for cows. On one occasion our ploughman asked me to buy him a copy of that week's *Truth*. It was my first contact with that extraordinary periodical. I spread it out on the handlebars on the way home. 'Muggins Mauls his Missus' said the headlines. I was less concerned about Muggins than about the editor. Surely he could never have been to a secondary school.

There were produced subtle changes in community life but the main engineer of change in the backblocks was probably Henry Ford. His little black box mounted on four skinny wheels caused town and country to shorten the bridge of time and distance so that they virtually overlapped. The early Ford was an engineering triumph. There was no battery, no self-starter, no petrol pump, no gears, no clutch, no dashboard, no panel of controls. It was in fact an automatic car, long before its time. When the pedal was out the car was in top. When it was pushed down the car was in low. Halfway (held temporarily by the foot and permanently by pulling on the hand-brake) was neutral. This was essential for starting. Otherwise the owner, cranking in front with the pedal out could be trampled to death. The pedal moved in a slot in the wooden floor and if the alignment was faulty the pedal tended to stick in low gear. The car then became a fearsome thing: an irresistible force plunging ahead in a search for an immovable object. Our car was thus afflicted before I chiselled some of the wood away. My father was never at home in the car. His skill was with horses. On one occasion he drove into the galvanized iron shed that was our garage and the car was stuck in low gear. I yelled, 'Get your toe behind it, pull it back.' He did not hear me for he was tugging at the wheel and shouting, 'Whoa, whoa'. The car responded, but not before it had passed through the garage wall into the hen run.

Those were the golden days of motoring. The car was an entirely new medium of transport and its ownership was as simple as its engine. There were no rules of the road except that it was courteous to keep to the left and it was wise to be cautious at intersections. There was no driving licence, no warrant of fitness, no parking restrictions, no petrol stations and practically no motoring offences. Instead was the open road, distance coming to meet us, the car hood down and the wind whistling the song of freedom, as in the short space of an hour we could cover a full twenty-five miles. Our car was originally intended to be a pleasure vehicle for my mother, and when the technique of lifting her in and out had been mastered, a true pleasure vehicle it became. But this did not stop it becoming a farm utility. Once we went to Christchurch. A later visit was to an aunt and uncle in Timaru. My uncle, Henry Faber-Brown, a gentleman and a conservative of the old school, walked round the car, touched the front tyres with the toe of his boot in order to prove reality and mused, 'D'you mean to say that that thing took you to Christchurch and back?' Indeed, given adequate petrol, oil, water, patience and luck it could have taken us to England and back. It was replaced many years later by another car, less efficient but more elegant. I think it possible that even now, though sixty years old, it may still be chugging away in the background of a saw bench, a milking machine or a pump.

Except for the chairmanship of the school committee there was no hierarchy in Fairview. Its residents were bound by a peasant-like egality and though differing violently among themselves on politics, religion and farming procedures they fully endorsed the right to differ. Apart from the socials and dances connected with the school prizes, the only other communal effort was the Mutual Improvement Society with (I think) monthly meetings each devoted to one of four special purposes. On the social evening the school room was comfortably filled with concert-goers and dancers. On the religious evening, usually taken by my father, there were never more than a faithful dozen. I forget the purpose of the other two evenings – possibly music and literature. It was a brave effort, a fore-runner of the W.E.A., but it was not a success. Fairview based its views on whims and prejudices and did not need mental exercises to confirm or refute them. This was well shown by any electioneering campaign. The candidate would arrive from Timaru, vehemently denunciate his political opponents, and leave expressing his confidence in the wisdom of Fairview. Half an hour later he would be repeating his act at Claremont, the next school.

He usually left chaos behind. Everyone wanted to be the first to contribute to the debate. As a result the only speakers that could be heard were those with the loudest voices. When my father was chairman he would insist vainly on the formalities of public meetings. The truth was that he was not politically acceptable to the majority. They did not approve of secondary education for his sons, nor his support for Ward rather than Massey. Ward was a good friend of the farmers but made little show of it, while Massey, being himself a farmer, was regarded as a rugged bulwark between the retention of private ownership of farms and the rapacities of socialism. But even more decisive was the Protestantism of Massey and the Catholicism of Ward. My father's political opponents were merciless in this. They insisted that only a hypocrite could profess Protestantism in the community and favour Catholicism in Parliament. Their vehemence tended to turn their views into political cudgels. I remember one weather-beaten little freeholder leaping on a back desk and shouting above the hubbub, 'Why did they paint the Temuka railway station green if it wasn't to please the Catholics?' I was very impressed at the sinister significance of this revelation. When my father snorted that they probably had a surplus of green paint I felt it was a weak reply. It is hard at the present day to explain this Catholic-Protestant enmity. Perhaps the prejudices of the Tudors and the Stuarts lived on. In 1879 an Orangeman's procession through the streets of Christchurch degenerated into a fight with Catholics. Why? I remember a wrestling match with my best friend at school. It had started playfully enough but each in turn got hurt and got angry. When I had a temporary ascendancy I used the cutting phrase 'Catholic pig' – at which he shot back with 'Protestant dog'. This shocked me. What right had the Catholics to regard us as we regarded them?

I have heard my grandfather say that in the very early days of Pleasant Valley nearly all the settlers on our side happened to be Catholics and on the other side Protestants. There was no importance in this coincidence until St Patrick's Day when the prudent stayed indoors and shots were fired across the valley. The next day all was peace and the kids returned to my grandmother's school. It is an improbable story as so many of my grandfather's were. Pleasant Valley is undoubtedly pleasant but it is not much of a valley. The story fails geographically. It also fails because it lacks all motivation.

Once on the Orari railway station my father watched one of his farming friends farewell his daughter who was *en route* to a convent in Christchurch. When the train had gone:

'Isn't she a saint, Bennett? Don't you think she is a saint?'

'She would be no less a saint if she married one of those chaps across the road and had a dozen kids.'

'If you were a younger man, Bennett, I'd give you a thick ear for that.'

'You couldn't get near my ear.'

'Off with your coat, Bennett.'

At this stage the station master intervened. He talked the enmity out of it and the friendship back.

I once heard my mother state that she would always prefer a good Catholic to a bad Protestant. This astonished me and for the first time I began to question her judgement. Perhaps she had not read *Westward Ho!*

All through our boyhood the shadow of my mother loomed. I am afraid our close association tended to dull our sympathy. We did not see then as we saw fifty years later the poignancy of some of her simple acts. There was for instance, the old black box. Every few months she would get one of us to turn out the old black box. It was of London origin, a massive structure of teak or sandalwood, tarred on the outside and faintly sticky through the decades. Inside was a miscellany of silks and satins, velvets and plush, lace, tape, spangles, tooled leather, tweeds and serge. This was the commercial residue of her dress-making days. One by one, at her command, we would pass each item to her and while she nursed and fingered it, we would be back in the book again. Then the article would be replaced perhaps in a different situation and another one passed up. We regarded it as a senseless whim. It never occurred to us that each article told a story and that all the stories were of youth and health. She also had a treasure book of pressed flowers – ferns, clovers, daisy petals. I know now that they were gathered not in Woodgreen, London, but in Pleasant Valley. There was also a croquet set, polished and complete. When her infirmity had anchored her firmly in her chair, she would allow us to take out one mallet, one ball and one hoop. Then, as new pains flared and hope dimmed she permitted us a wider choice until finally we helped ourselves and left the pieces to disintegrate out in the weather. I used to leave a mallet under the monkey puzzle tree on the front lawn. Last year I visited the place. The monkey puzzle tree was still there. So also might have been the rotting shape of the croquet mallet. But I had not the heart to look. At the time it all represented eccentricities. Now it illustrates the tragedy of a young bride, deeply in love and therefore confident of everything, going to the country of which she knew nothing, taking the black box whose contents would allow her to do fancy dressmaking to the astonishment of her husband. She would lead a lady's life which included some genteel croquet with neighbours. She also developed the hobby of searching the Pleasant Valley road for fancies in floral design. And with never a thought in 1897 of rheumatoid arthritis.

My mother's illness, of course, invited every resource of therapy.

Though the pathology had been accepted as the will of the Lord, yet there was always a feeling that the Lord might have made a mistake, an administrative bungle, so to speak, and so, without impiety, all other methods could be explored. An itinerant hot gospeller once discovered her hobbling painfully from room to room. He knew nothing of rheumatism but was a specialist in faith. 'You haven't enough faith, you are relying on your crutches. Burn your crutches. If you had faith as a grain of mustard seed [which though Biblical is a meaningless phrase]. Burn your crutches.' So she burned her crutches and never walked again.

For her, medicines were soon exhausted. A country practitioner gave her a course of useless injections. The surgeons who removed her appendix straightened her knees under the anaesthetic and left her in acute misery for the next two years. For some weeks a self-described nurse lived in the house. She was untrained, devout, spectacularly arrayed in a purple and white uniform and confident of her mastery of rheumatism. After a series of 'treatments' which seemed without purpose or result my father demanded an explanation of her rationale. She replied that she approached each day with an open mind and did as the Lord directed. The Lord then directed my father to put her and her box in the trap and deliver them both that afternoon to Timaru.

Then followed the hot air treatment. Her legs, swaddled in masses of wrappings, were extended to fit into a metal cradle, covered with a metal lid, the whole raised on supports. It was then heated from below by a heater dependent on vaporised kerosene. It was a monster of a device. To start it, two ingredients were required – methylated spirits and patience. My father had little of the latter and often an awesome geyser of flame hit the ceiling. The patient was supposed to endure the maximum heat for as long as possible which gave no safety margin when the patient could make no adjustments herself. It was distressing, dangerous and utterly ineffective.

The beef treatment came next, backed by a badly written book with a title something like 'How to get well and keep well'. The basis of the treatment was topside beef. No other cut would do. It was bought fresh minced, put in a pot with a little water, which had then to be placed in a larger pot of boiling water and then kept simmering for hours. The final product was composed of tough gelatinous lumps, covered by a grey sludge. It was not only uninviting, it was repulsive. Yet this was my mother's exclusive diet for nearly three years. Only occasionally and then most guiltily would she yield to a crust or a segment of apple. Surprisingly her general health did not appear to suffer. She should have been wrecked by a range of vitamin deficiencies but as far as I remember was not. How wisely does nature adjust to the foolishness of man. How foolishly does man pretend to correct the dietetic clumsiness of nature.

The years passed. There was a period with herbs, longer periods with faith healing or spiritual healing in a variety of forms. There was a correspondence with Ratana . . . . Finally, with all hope exhausted there came resignation and with resignation some easing of the pain.

Inexorably the disease broke her physically but it never crushed her spirit. I have told elsewhere of her war labours (in *The Tenth Home* Auckland, Blackwood and Janet Paul, 1966). The war asked for money and goods from civilians. My father gave one of his best horses which deserved a better fate than dying at sea or in France. My mother had nothing to give except the painful labours of her twisted hands and for this she selected the Belgian refugees: clad in rags, stiff with cold, blue-fingered babies in a white landscape. She found a few garments, explored again the black box, and made us push her chair to the sewing machine. My father bought material as she ordered. Friends brought her minor rolls of cotton, of wool and of flannelette. Doggedly she kept at it as her joints permitted. The machine was worked reluctantly by one of her sons who would sprawl on the floor with one hand on the spindle of the flywheel, eyes, of course, deep in a book and responding reflexly to her orders, 'Go . . . slow . . . fast . . . just as you like . . . slow . . . stop'. My father, enjoined to find a suitable container (no cartons in those days) came home with a tea-chest the volume of which was probably a cubic yard. He offered to cut it down to any size she wanted but she accepted the challenge and the planned campaign of a few weeks extended into more than two years. The stiff fingers pushed and guided the fabric beneath the tread of the needle. Laboriously she made button holes and sewed on buttons. At length her triumph was assured. The tea-chest was full, pressed down and still full. Another garment, said my father, and it could not be nailed down. So she desisted. Her sons got up off the floor. The chest was closed, addressed, taken to Timaru and handed over to the authorities. There was little security in those days and we were aware of the vessel in which it left New Zealand. Half-way on its voyage the vessel was sunk. My father said nothing, which was at least a positive reaction for there was nothing to say. 'It is the will of the Lord,' said my mother, her voice trembling. I remember thinking savagely that if she were correct then the Lord must have been deep in with the Germans.

About 1910 a bike accident left me with a fractured humerus and clavicle and these had to be submitted to X-ray on three consecutive days before Dr Unwin was satisfied. It was taken in a two-storeyed building in the lower end of North Street which is now the Timaru Electric Institute. The radiographer was an elderly man who, I seem to remember, had had something to do with the Timaru Post Office. The service was available only for a short period of each day when the power was on. I was given to understand, though I cannot confirm it, that this was very early in the history of X-rays in Timaru and preceded any hospital X-ray. Apart from the pain and discomfort of much arm-manipulation with no anaesthetic, the gratifying side-effects included the deference of the school to one who had actually survived an X-ray and had acquired an ostentatious plaster. The only exception was my brother, who had to milk the cows for the next few weeks.

In the early hours of one morning my father dragged me from bed to see Halley's comet. 'You'll never see it again,' but he might be wrong. There out over the sea about five miles beyond Timaru, though the astronomers insisted on five million miles, was a great golden object passing from south to north in a low arc above the horizon. (Again I have to differ from the astronomers about the direction.) What appeared to be the tail fanned out in the south like the spangles of a fireworks rocket. A patient of the present day recounted how she saw it, probably on that same night, from the ferry on its way to Lyttelton; a Maori football team on board was confident that the end of the world had come. This was a common belief everywhere. The comet was regarded as a portent of disaster, the more so as King Edward had died a few days before. Also on the ferry was a Salvation Army band which held other views on the end of the world and went on playing lustily.

I remember my father's intense interest in the Johnson Jeffries' heavyweight championship, the apprehension over Powelka and the sensation of Amy Bock who married one of her own sex. ('But how?' I was genuinely puzzled. 'I mean . . . .' 'It's not worth discussing,' my mother assured me with an emphasis which closed the subject.) I knew from listening to my parents the broad outlines of the Hall murder in Timaru, even though it had happened twenty years before. In 1913 there was intense public interest in the great General Strike. All the farmers with more buoyancy than was appropriate to the issues rallied behind Massey and his special constables and generally approved their excesses. To them the clothing retailer (Thomson, was it?) who, riding on a donkey led the procession of volunteer labour down to the ships, was an undoubted hero.

Saturday was sale day. Nearly always our trap had some saleable produce under the seat. My father always came home full of his adventures which he would retail to us at the meal table. The meal was almost invariably fish which he had purchased at the wharf and which I had insisted on frying. My mother so repeatedly praised my ability as a

70

fish-frier that I, a veritable Simple Simon, would not admit any rival near the stove. Under the wharf where the fish was sold was an old eccentric endlessly manipulating sheets of iron, spouting and wire in an attempt to harness the waves. A few well-wishers gave him odd coins. Among these was my father whose motives were sympathy and whose excuse was, 'You never can tell'.

Occasionally we too would go into town in the trap and would be dismissed with a shilling each. Most of this went in a fish shop in (I think) Sophia Street. It was the sort of place where instead of a meal one got a feed: an enormous fried flounder, none too clean, and piles of buttered bread. This cost ninepence each, which seems so incredible, even for those days, that we might have been charged at half rates for children. But when the price went up to a shilling we were outraged. This meant living from hand to mouth. So we boycotted the shop and were somewhat surprised that it still kept in business.

In high school days life was mainly a grey routine. A scramble to get to school on time, total involvement with classes, games and sport and the long trudge home to the cows often with a nor'-wester contesting every revolution of the pedals. Opposite the beginning of our farm lived a family, the Squires, whose daughter had gone for a year or more to the Girls' School. She would cement our academic bond by shouting as I passed 'Parleyvoo Frongsay?' and I would reply loudly and inaccurately 'Oui, oui'. Such conversations greatly impressed her father, who regarded them as dividends on his outlay. After a year or so the dialogue broke down. She was probably forgetting her vocabulary.

Yet it was a grand stretch of country between Cicero at one end and the cows at the other. Far to the west the Alps became mobile, folding the sun away for the day. Shapes and shadows merged on the flat landscape, as if the lights in the auditorium were dimmed and beneath the nor'-west arch the pastel colours moved with the precision of slow ballet. Not an artist's country, this, but a poet's. Always there is poetry in every sky bridging earth and space.

Somewhere during the course of the war my father developed a crippling arthritis. The acute stages lasted about a year but a chronic stage, apparently permanent, followed. Half the farm, on which was the extra house, was sold. The ploughman went and so did the maid, the latter being irreplaceable during the war. The main responsibility of the farm fell on me, with three younger brothers, all at school, in support. I was continually asking my father's advice and continually being told to use my own judgement. The farm barely survived and then only because of the firmer prices during the war. Still doggediy patriotic, we grew wheat at a loss. Then my father improved a little and began to appear at times in the yard. But it seemed to me that he would never farm again, and this left me little option. I had just passed Matriculation and the time seemed suitable. I went to tell him that I was not going back to school and he could now count on me all the year round. He was out beyond the yard gate, leaning on a stick and slashing at thistles with a sickle. He heard me out (it was a pretty speech, not altogether unrehearsed) and then said I was a silly young fool, that I was being given a chance which neither he nor anyone else in the district had had and that I was to get back to my books. He then turned his back on me and went on swiping at thistles.

My protests were genuine for I was truly concerned about him. But for myself the protests had no great depth. As my responsibilities on the farm had broadened so had my conviction that farming was not for me. Something repelled me. I did not know then what it was but I know now. It was the unremitting involvement with farm animals, the wretched piteous dumb animals. I have seen a horse zigzagging up a hill with a fat man sitting on the shaft, lambs dying in a blizzard, thirsty horses denied a minute for drinking in mid-stream, kittens tied in a sugar bag with stones and tossed into the dam, a horse-collar strapping down a shoulder ulcer, dogs tied up for three days without food. I have used a whip on horses, have killed sheep and pigs and hens, have shot a cow with a gangrenous udder, have helped to tail and castrate lambs, have milked through several seasons a frantic kicking cow without suspecting its tuberculous udder, have delivered a mare with obstructed neck presentation, have watched the agonies of a dog dying from strychnine, and because I was too weak to step out of the fashion of the day I have shot ducks and rabbits and hares in the name of sport.

I hated every minute of it.

'But animals don't feel,' say the gallants in red coats whose dogs tear a hare to pieces. Animals do feel. The same pain-receptive neurological structures existing in man also exist in animals. Only in intelligence are they not comparable. Many of their diseases have the same pathology. When the crushing pain of a coronary thrombosis grips a man it has a funereal ring. He stops in his tracks, frightened to move. He is treated in an intensive-care ward with rest and nursing and drugs and automatic alarms. When a horse is arrested with a coronary thrombosis his heart falters and he is treated with the whip. Some day a new generation will demand reform and when that day comes no animals will be killed for food while in a conscious state, and no dehorning, no docking and no castration will be done without an anaesthetic. 'Impossible,' say those who have no technical knowledge and no imagination.

So I went back to school for another two years. My conscience about the farm eased as my father improved and my brother, third in the family, abandoned a secondary education and worked tirelessly on the farm until he incurred rheumatic fever. These last two years were spent in the élite University Scholarship class of seven. Two gained scholarships. I had to be content with a credit pass which was a deep disappointment for my effort had been almost maximal. My parents were staunchly consoling. 'Those scholarship winners,' said my mother. 'Can any of them milk a cow?' 'Or build a stack?' added my father. I neither knew nor cared. The point at issue was a scholarship.

I left school with guarded optimism. Within a year it had all been crushed out of me. I was back home, desultorily working on the farm, or on neighbours' farms, a University drop-out with no ambition, no future.

And as if to offset the banal placidity of the cud-chewing cows I determined on my future.

I would enlist and go to the war.

The motives needed no excuse. The Goth was at the gate, the country was in peril, England and also Fairview expected every man to do his duty. There was no doubt of the German atrocities; they were always being confirmed in the *Timaru Herald*. Patriotism was the pure motive and thereafter any right thinking man had no option. But the initial steps were not easy. I could not enlist without my parents' consent. 'Your mother will never agree,' warned my father. 'Your father will never consent,' insisted my flabbergasted mother. I set to work on them. It was not hard to break my father. I threatened to run away from home as he and his father had done and enlist under a false name. Secretly I think this pleased him. But my mother withstood some weeks of rather brutal pressure before she gave in and tremulously signed the form. Then came boarding and attestation. All I remember of the boarding was marching in the nude up and down the Timaru drill hall while two medical officers on all fours studied my feet. When they rose one said, ' 'Fraid you're grade four, laddie. Flattest feet I've ever seen.'

I had never heard of flat feet. I regarded the diagnosis as an insult and exploded indignantly. I had played football, had always run the full course in steeplechases, had followed a team all day . . . my feet were as good as any in the countryside. I demanded a reconsideration. I was much worked up and this (and silent reading) had inspired me with fluency. They listened in genuine surprise and then conferred. 'All right then. We'll make you grade one and you can steeplechase in the trenches. And don't blame me if you get killed.'

Half an hour later we were taking the oath. We sat, a dozen or so, on forms round three sides of a bare room. In the centre was a table at which sat the attesting officer, a peppery little first lieutenant. His head deep in papers he would call the next name and the man would stand across the table from him.

'Put your hand on the Bible. Repeat what I say. I swear by Almighty God . . . .'

The man ahead of me was a gangling youth, almost certainly a country product. As he finished, something made the officer look up. He burst into a torrent of invective. 'What the bloody hell do you mean taking the oath with your hat on?' The wretched youth snatched his hat off but the tirade continued. I was aghast. It was no way for gentlemen to converse. 'You'll have to take the damn thing again. Put your hand on the Bible. No – not there, you can't use that again.' He flicked over the polluted page to the New Testament, which apparently could guarantee a more binding military allegiance.

Later I collected my first day's military pay, a postal note for five shillings, and went home, a certified soldier of the King.

5

The War Afar Off

The troop train paused impatiently at the Timaru Station and on the platform were N.C.O.s calling names. I bade farewell to my distraught mother, sitting bolt upright on the front seat of the Ford, and shook hands with my father. His firm and lingering grip was the only advice he gave me, but I knew what he meant. I grinned and nodded at my brothers and they grinned and nodded back. I suspect the Ford nodded too. It would now be driven more gently.

Deflation started about Temuka. The obese gent sitting opposite me with the slurred voice and the beer-stained waistcoat pointed out that I was an intruder in a carriage full of soldiers who were going to fight and almost certainly die for the likes of me. When my turn came I would understand this. He let me stay but insisted that I remember . . . that I remember . . . apparently it was something that he couldn't remember. And the only other thing that I do remember was that he deserted at Christchurch.

The deflation accelerated on the ship to Wellington. At 5 p.m. we were secured on board with guards on the gangways. We were assigned a hold in the stern over the propeller. Round the perimeter were three-tiered bunks and in the centre some mess tables and forms without backs. There we were shortly served our first army meal: thick slices of mutton, with boiled potatoes and liberal supplies of tomato and Worcestershire sauce. Round me were men nearly twice my age, friendly, and almost forcing me to become involved in the conversation. The theme seemed to be the weather. It was going to be a dirty night, heaven help the seasick, lucky we were to have plenty of Worcester sauce to prevent it. Was it any good, I asked? Any good? It was the perfect answer, lad. Nothing else was any good. I was grateful and poured more on my plate, mashed up another potato with it. Nice chaps, so helpful. I went up on deck and stayed till we were at sea. It was my first voyage. Near the Lyttelton Heads the vessel twice stumbled and went down on its knees. I began to wonder whether I had overdone the Worcester sauce. Down in the hold the air was grey with tobacco smoke, and nauseous with beer. At the tables were now a number of noisy poker schools. I clambered to my bunk and before I could lie down I groped for my strawberry box.

That interminable night carried us north on leaden feet. After a time the poker players had gone, the lights were out, the rumble of the screw rose and fell, the ship staggered and reeled and from the bunks came moans and groans and sudden explosive sounds.

Eventually, as if several weeks later, the ship became motionless and I had my first view of Wellington, windy, wet, drained and yet colourful. We were a silent group. The night had buried the Worcester sauce joke. Though I still reeled I probably maintained a little of my patriotism, but the Empire I was going to defend was now a flabby affair.

We got to the station and were formed into a wavering line. There was a roll call. Then came an obese corporal, tugging a trolly. To each man he gave a large tin pannikin of coffee, strong, sweet and hot. It was nectar indeed. As we sipped it the marine insults of the night were forgotten and replaced by the reassuring solidity of land. One effect of the coffee was to remind us of the emptiness of our stomachs. Whereupon our corporal went down the line again helping each man to a huge mutton sandwich. It had plenty of butter, plenty of salt and Worcester sauce, was inelegant and wholly satisfactory. The British Empire came into closer focus. Perhaps the British were not such fools for being a maritime power. We ate the last crumbs, handed back the empty pannikins to the corporal – if this was his war effort how magnificent it was – and boarded the train for Trentham.

It was all noise, noise, noise to one who had never met men in the mass before. The clamour of the camp had a martial raucousness in all its variations; a company of men marching in hobnailed boots, the stentorian voices of sergeants drilling squads, a band leading a parade, whistles as time signals, 'Order arms' and the crash of rifle butts, trucks lumbering familiarly about the camp, the rattle of distant rifle fire, the bugle signing the day off with the moving Retreat, the night torn apart by the sanitary squad slamming their buckets about, the imperious summons of the Reveille to another day.

Infantry training was robot-like stuff, asking more of the feet than the brain. I slid into its easy routine, so much less strenuous than a day in the harvest paddock. I enjoyed the recreation huts in the evening, wrote home frequently and worked away at physics for the special exam in Wellington. I would be informed of the date, said the New Zealand University, and I duly was, two days after the exam had been held. The University, long since defunct, still owes me two guineas. The only incident of note concerned my big toe, injured while harvesting and after ten days in Trentham an excruciating infected mass under the tight constriction of heavy hobnailed army boots. The pain one day anchored me in a drill movement and the drill sergeant, a specialist in malingering, reported me to our company commander who was passing. I overheard some of their conversation. 'Refusing to obey lawful horder, sir.' 'If you order him to do something he can't do, Sergeant, then your order isn't lawful.' 'No sir, yes sir.' I was handed to the medical officer whose diagnosis of the toe was: 'That's a mess'. He gave me the precious slip to D. and T. (excused duty, and treatment which was heavy quantities of boracic ointment and pink lint). After ten days the nail came off and the boot went on and I limped back to the parade ground.

Every month a new reinforcement was called up, trained for a little over two months, sent on final leave for ten days, reassembled, issued with sea-kit, marched to Wellington and packed up into transports, while another motley crowd of civilians with overcoats and suitcases and sugar bags straggled through the camp gate. The 36ths were shaping up. We were as good as need be in all the bull-ring stuff, could manipulate a .303 with reasonable accuracy, had exhausted all the resources of the Trentham trenches, had charged and plunged our bayonets into Teutonic sacks of straw, finishing each movement with a grunt and a twist of the bayonet. We had endured lengthy route marches and finished each day with P.T. Because the dread cerebro-spinal meningitis of the previous year could return there were regular preventative potassium permanganate gargles. The pinkish purple fluid was carried on to the parade ground in buckets and we filed past, each man filling his tin pannikin, and then in small groups gargling round the waste buckets. Some of the men drank it, either to save time or to flout authority. Its efficacy was minimal whatever the route.

Every evening Routine Orders were posted. This extraordinary publication with its cryptic abbreviations, its special vocabulary, its unemotional declarations, interested me as a new literary device. It represented the mechanism by which the hierarchy of the army rose and fell. After a time I lost interest. Then one evening, on the advice of a tent-mate I examined the current issue at first curiously and then incredulously. There was my name correct in spelling, in initials and in regimental number. And it went on to inform everyone in Trentham Camp that I was promoted to the rank of lance-corporal.

It is the greatest rank in the army, that of lance-corporal. He has been singled out, a person with unique qualities. All subsequent promotions are merely matters of degree. The basic essentials have been defined by that first rank.

I procured a single stripe, and sewed it on with great care, heavy thread and an excess of stitches. It looked splendid. But no one cheered. No one commented. Indifference permeated the camp like a fog. But a few days later when the whistle blew for the end of the training period and the sergeant who was drilling our small squad said to me, 'March 'em off, Corporal, and dismiss'. So I stepped out and with appropriate orders marched 'em off. There was no argument. They dutifully responded. And why not? My authority, given a little devious logic, could probably be traced back to War Cabinet, London.

The glow persisted for over a week and then came that fateful day when I was mess orderly. To the other seven occupants of our bell-tent I bore back at midday the standard loaf of bread, slab of butter, tin of jam and dixie of tea. My mates received the ration with scorn. There was no bonus of pickles or cheese, and the jam was the old tasteless mush with the whimsical label of plum and apple. Surely I could do better than that? Where was the resource that a corporal was supposed to have? In the cookhouse, I was reminded, were rows and rows of the delectable melon and ginger jam. Anyone with a swift approach and a bit of courage could effect an exchange. 'Nothing in it Corporal.'

I took the tin back and after a flank approach stepped round the corner and made a swift exchange. I was almost clear when the sergeant cook came charging out. He was greasy, obese, angry, intolerant and insulting. He refused to accept my story of an exchange, although when he relieved me of the melon and ginger he let me take a plum and apple substitute. I gave him my name and number which is all that is required of a P.O.W. He was going to lay an orderly-room charge, he said. I returned disconsolately to the tent. One of the men stood up. He came from the same town as the sergeant cook and he knew something of his past. He went off confidently but after a time came back slowly, his eyes on the ground. It turned out that the cook, surprisingly, knew something about him. My friend regretted that my case would not be helped if he and the cook laid down their cards.

In the end there was no orderly-room charge but the orderly-room advised that the Company Commander wished to see me. He was a pleasant, affable person, who in civilian life could easily have been president of an Old Boys' Club. 'What's this I hear, Bennett? Wholesale purloining of His Majesty's stores.' I launched into emphatic defence. He seemed to derive amusement from my earnestness. (I was to learn later that my crime is the sort that is condoned provided no one forces the issue.) Then he said:

'I've been looking up your personal file. You're a medical student, I believe. You should be in the medical corps.'

'No, Sir.' This was frightening. I was a medical student only in name. I wanted to remain in a combatant unit. I had just finished my infantry training. I had no liking, no aptitude for the medical corps . . . .

'A good soldier, Corporal, goes where he is sent. He also takes what he is given even if it is only plum and apple. All right, you may go.'

Three days later I had an exclusive portion of Routine Orders to myself. '74420 L/cpl. F. O. Bennett reverts to the rank of Pte, is posted to N.Z. Med. Corps and is transferred to Awapuni Camp.'

I protested of course – with more emphasis than was wise. It was soon obvious that though a good soldier goes where he is sent, a protesting one is sent where someone of rank thinks he ought to go.

The difference between Trentham and Awapuni reflected the difference between the science of killing and the art of saving. The trenches, rifles and bayonets were replaced by stretchers, splints, bandages, surgical haversacks, artificial respiration and fireman's lift. The standards of ceremonial drill and military decorum were set higher in Awapuni. Every night the guard was inspected before being posted and the best-dressed man was given leave. Although this was a lean bait (for Awapuni Camp in the evening had far more diversions than had the dim streets of Palmerston North) yet there was intense competition for the distinction. There were many lectures usually from sergeants of the permanent staff. They taught us little. The evacuation of the wounded was, we were told, by the maltese cart. We scorned this and our sergeant agreed that though stretcher-bearers were now substituted, he had to teach what was laid down. We laboriously learned all the pressure points for stopping arterial haemor-rhage (an armchair teaching of no practical use). We were more proficient in the bones of the body than in the treatment of any of the fractured.

The hospital for Awapuni Camp was at the Racecourse, Featherston. It was mostly empty and though we spent nearly a month there we were never once inside it. Instead lectures were substituted mostly from the Officer Commanding, Major Little, an elderly amiable Scot who had been a general practitioner in Timaru. He had no syllabus and lectured where his whim led, usually on erudite clinical matters as if to advanced medical students. He spent much time on syphilis, especially syphilis of the third stage. Tabes in the army would be as much an anachronism as would bow and arrow. The one word that was best remembered was 'phlebitis': the meaning was forgotten but the sound was amusing.

There were also many lectures from sergeants on hygiene and sanitation and every Saturday morning there was a long written examination. I worked hard at these seeing a possible way to get back my stripe. It became apparent later that the purpose of the exams was to keep us busy while the sergeants prepared for weekend leave. Our papers went to the incinerator without being read.

I had now dropped three months and was in the 39th reinforcements.

One lived with one's mates more intimately in Awapuni than in Trentham. There were many conscientious objectors with beliefs that might be religious or political or ethical or personal. There was a diverting number of cranks, such as those who were violent in their opposition to violence, or the man who had a vision that his real name was John the Disciple of the Lord and refused to sign his paybook otherwise, or the man who insisted on a beard till we held him down and shaved the left half of his face. Some were attracted to the medical corps because of a sense of mission, others because of an erroneous belief that it was safer. The true conscientious objectors, though in a minority, set a high standard of work and discipline and the army owed them much. The rest were a more earthy type drafted for no special reason into the medical corps. Here, as in Trentham, there were many who accepted their posting without question, claiming that one part of the bloody army was the same as any other part of the bloody army and that everyone above the rank of private was a bastard and there you were.

The army can be a lonely place unless one has a special confidant whose friendship is loyal and instinctive. My special buddy was John Nagle. He had been a steel worker in Sheffield a decade or more before. Now he was making coal ranges in Napier or Gisborne. He was big, slow-speaking, with a Midlands accent. The only quality we had in common was friendship. He was more than twice my age and we differed over politics, religion, patriotism, alcohol, women, the character of sergeants, and the sanity of officers. Our opinions were in such contrast that we ploughed a good deal of the comic into our debates and when there could have been asperity there was only amusement. He was no great soldier, old John, lacking aggressiveness, and I was no great soldier, lacking maturity, but either would have gone to the endurable limit in defence of the other. There has never been any satisfactory analysis of friendship. There need not be. Like gravity, it is intangible, invisible and mighty.

One day a Medical Officer said to me, 'This fellow Nagle that you get around with – what's he after?' I was completely puzzled. I knew of nothing he was after. 'Well,' said the officer awkwardly dismissing the subject, 'Don't let things go too far.' It was not till long after that I realized what he meant and at the same time realized how wrong he had been.

In the medical corps we wore a flamboyant red cross on the left arm. It had replaced my single stripe and I hated it. I did not know then that the only two men who had won a V.C. and bar had been medical officers, nor that the third was to be a Canterbury farmer. Particularly did I resent my status of medical student. No one could have deprecated more than I did the sole achievement of an Intermediate pass in Chemistry. My protests were useless. Before long I was called tn at times to assist in the First Aid Post. Actually it was an easy job. The man with trouble in his chest got the black medicine. The man with a bellyache got the white medicine which always had to be shaken first. The man with the wrong diagnosis got the wrong medicine but seemed none the worse. I was once consulted by a stranger from another company. He had slept in after Reveille and had been forced to take the dangerous escape route of claiming to be sick. He was now about to confront a suspicious Medical Officer, 'Say, digger, you're a medical student aren't you? Know any decent symptoms?'

The 36ths were leaving New Zealand. The infantry that day would swing down to Wellington and tomorrow would be at sea. And I would have been with them had it not been for a tin of plum and apple jam. In Awapuni the 36ths were broken up into squads of a dozen or so, each squad to travel 'on duty' on a transport. When the last group was within a few hours of entraining they were two men short. Volunteers were called. Three men stepped out and two were selected. We disposed of our palliasses, received some inoculations and were issued with sea-kit, and finally reviewed by the Adjutant, a small efficient humourless officer who had lost an arm at Mons. At first he passed me, then looked over his shoulder and came back. 'How old are you? Where do you come from? Have you had any final leave? Does your mother know you're sailing tomorrow?' Then with a nonchalance I thought outrageous he said to the orderly officer, 'Fall this man out. Get someone else from Details.'

I fell out, handed my sea-kit in again and went back to my humble corner in the 39ths. It was hardly worth trying.

Near the end of our training the great Raetihi bush fires occurred. One mid-morning a great black curtain came rolling down from the north and engulfed us. Almost as quickly came the rumour of a volcanic eruption. Visibility was a few yards only and in the buildings candles were lit. Two companies of the 39ths were paraded for duty. We were issued with two water bottles per man, a surgical haversack each, heavy supplies of picric acid and a cloth for the face. We spent the day resoaking our puttees and waiting for orders. When the order came it was to dismiss.

It is almost impossible to keep out of trouble in the army. One Saturday I was in Palmerston North, miserable with toothache. My upper teeth had many gaps and there was much dental caries. I decided, knowing nothing about it, that they were not worth saving. I marched into a civilian dentist and requested him to take the upper ones out. This he did and charged me one pound. Next morning, utterly miserable, I went on sick parade to try and avoid church parade. The Medical Officer exploded at my audacity in thinking I had any say regarding my teeth. They were the property of His

Majesty's Government whose executive officers belonged to the Dental Corps. When he ran out of invective he put me on L.D. (Light Duty). The orderly sergeant, always in trouble over Sunday fatigues, marked me down immediately for telephone duty, and I sat for eight hours in a draughty box receiving and directing the outside calls. By the end of the duty I was in a treacherous mood, still loyal to the Empire, but not to all its components. Then the phone rang. A harsh voice said:

'Is that the camp? Butcher here. How many sausages d'you want in the morning?'

'How many did you send last week?'

He named some quantity.

'Well, it wasn't enough,' (which was true). 'We want double the quantity tomorrow,' (untrue).

'You want . . . what?' His voice was rising.

'Double the quantity,' I said firmly.

'Gawd!' Then after a pause:

'All right, boss, I'll see what I can do.'

The next morning there was a glut. Some men had six. Everyone had their fill except I, their benefactor, who could not bite.

Final leave was a flop. I slept the journey down on a hatch, which seemed the only way to get pure air. At home they did not know what to do with me, except that I was not to do any work. I did milk a few cows with a certain satisfaction, despite the family's disapproval. 'What are you going to do today?' my mother would ask, determined to turn every minute into an asset. There was little to do. I called on a few neighbours who were effusive enough but were too busy to make an occasion of it. There was a visit to the High School, a hearty farewell from Mr Thomas, and his selection of the traditional three books from Huttons to be entered on his account. Fairview provided the standard social and dance in my honour. At the end of the social the chairman presented me with a wrist-watch with name and number engraved. He said that he was sure they would all agree that the honour of Fairview was et cetera et cetera and the honour-bearer replied that he could only promise to do his best et cetera et cetera. Then the pianist struck a chord, forms were swept back against the walls, the M.C. mounted a chair and no one thereafter gave a thought to the honour of Fairview.

Parting was not pleasant. My mother was convinced she was never going to see me again. I felt this was the wrong note. It was almost a pleasure to get back to camp. A new reinforcement was timidly picking its way about. Familiar faces increased as the trains came in. John Nagle, grinning, came round the corner. Having no relatives he had spent his leave in Wellington hotels, 'bar-bound' as he described it. I described it otherwise.

'There you go, lad, picking on a fellow again, the moment you see him. Bloody little nark you are. Can you lend me a quid?'

At sea with the wind rising and the *Tofua* beginning to toss. She was a small, compact transport, once in the island banana trade and now carrying infantry, divisional signallers and thirteen members of the medical corps.

The ship was full of strange noises and, among them, someone calling my name. The Medical Officer wanted me to report at the First Aid Post. He was young, smooth-faced and pleasant. 'I've arranged for you to be transferred here. You're a medical student aren't you? Give me a hand setting up this chair.'

It was a dental chair. We worked at it for a while and then he said, 'You all right?' I was surprised. Yes, of course I was all right. He tightened another nut and put the spanner down. 'I think I'll go below for a little.' He did not reappear for a week. I was tougher stuff. I reappeared after five days. During that time the ship was a shambles. Parade calls were not answered, meals were not eaten, rules and regulations were flouted. The discipline became more ragged and was finally jettisoned when one man, lying in bed pyjama-clad, turned a bleary eye on the master and said, 'For God's sake, Captain, stop this bloody boat.' He was, said an M.O., too ill to stand any punitive measures. Thereafter our sleeping quarters were exempt from inspection and gratefully we clutched and reeled on our way down below.

When after a week the storm was behind us and the ship had a recognizable routine I confided in my Medical Officer that my academic achievements went no further than terms in Physics and a pass in Chemistry. This did not deter him. He was in no mood to insist on high standards.

Fremantle in the evening, and thin lights and jagged shadows on the wharves. General leave was limited in time and space, and was in fact limited to one place which was the spacious reception quarters of the Perth Red Cross. This was my first of many encounters with this magnificent organization. It seemed to have unlimited quantities of the right food for famished soldiers. I ate shamelessly of cucumber and tomato sandwiches. Later I went on to the station hoping to get a quick run up to Perth. The military police thought otherwise. Australia, which had no conscription and was indifferent to deserters, was out of bounds to all New Zealand troops.

After Fremantle the troops were vaccinated against smallpox. It was an ill-timed procedure. There were no life-boats on board, merely stacks of rafts, and if a man had to swim for a raft he needed two active arms. (In the Second War the vaccinations were all completed in New Zealand.) My share in this was to mount guard on the deck over the newly vaccinated and to prevent them licking the lymph off before it dried.

Our therapeutic range in the First Aid Post was limited to three liniments, three ointments, about eight stock medicines and nine pills, including the notorious number nine. There were also a number of mysterious bottles in a locked cupboard with no available key.

Under my M.O.'s benign supervision I dressed septic ulcers, syringed ears, even did a few vaccinations. On a top shelf were a few medical text books, extraordinarily frank in their pictures. I thumbed these over and persuaded myself that I was doing a mini-medical course.

John Nagle and I leaning over the rail:

'The sea never changes,' said John. 'Same now as when I came out. Same waves going t'same way. See that albatross over there? Same bird I saw ten years ago.'

'That albatross is a seagull.'

'A common mistake, lad, first time at sea. But you'll learn.'

'And when you came out you went the other way. That bird must have hopped over Africa.'

'Oh, they get about. Got wings and things.'

He was a master of the absurd, John Nagle. In our arguments he made shameless use of his age. He was always referring to his experiences before I was born.

'Has nothing ever happened to you since?'

'Plenty. But I can't tell you. You might talk in your sleep.'

'Tell me, John. When did you leave home?'

'Afore you were born, lad.'

The inevitable boredom on a troopship was intensified on ours by regulations. No man during the hours of daylight was allowed to go below. He had to remain on deck, wet or fine, and there was no seating accommodation other than hatches and capstans. We also had to do without organized sport, games, recreation, space, fresh water for ablutions, shaving or showering. There was no beer, no gambling, no library, no group activities because of lack of room. On the other hand there was a daily newspaper composed of radio gleanings which could be read in a few minutes. A ship's magazine was produced. The infantry had regular rifle practice, firing at kerosene tins bobbing in the wake. Church parade was held every Sunday, during which the more distant rows of the congregation played poker.

There were of course some hotheads on board and a dangerous situation developed. The contrast between the privileges of officers and the limitations of the other ranks was too great. If a sweating soldier wanted a drink he got some tepid rusty water in a tin pannikin. If an officer wanted a drink he pressed a bell on the promenade deck (out of bounds to us). Later a steward would pick his way through men lying on the deck carrying aloft a tray of iced alcholic beverages. After a while the density of men round the companionway increased. The steward had to go warily and again and again caught the toe of one foot against the heel of another and lost control of his tray. After a while the technique changed. There may have been a bar on the promenade deck. The drinks probably flowed as freely but down a different channel.

Ship's regulations stipulated that there was to be no gambling. Yet the officers in the saloon, also out of bounds, gambled the day away. Then someone, never identified, but rumoured to be a padre, crept up to the saloon below the levels of the windows, then stood up and snapped. It was a splendid photo. Half the officers were there, all identifiable, sleeves rolled up, cards in hand, stacks of money on the side. Copies began to flood the ship. Batmen were always finding them in officers' quarters and asking what they should do with them.

In a war of propaganda it was a magnificent victory. Poker schools began to appear on hatchways and the kitty would always be built up on the exposed photo. Two-up and housie were soon openly operating. The favourite was Crown and Anchor and at least four boards flourished, the proprietors having obviously come prepared. To all this the officer strolling past was blind.

The small medical contingent also improved the amenities. There were two superstructures on the stern. One was our hospital and the other, about twelve feet square, was a mystery. No one knew what it contained and on ship's inspection the Master and the Officer Commanding Troops passed it by. Various attempts were made to pick the lock. Then, on the top of a medicine cabinet I found a key that fitted. Inside were some massive wooden crates marked: 'Comforts for troops on voyage'. But there was enough bare floor space to accommodate six palliasses. So six of us moved in and set up rules, blackouts and signals. We investigated the cases, probably there through several voyages, and found biscuits, sweets, tinned fruit, games, cards and magazines. We began distributing them among the troops, but this was risky. The job was taken over by an energetic little Y.M.C.A. padre, the same who had rolled up his sleeves and trouser legs and led the attack on the shambles of our hold after the first week at sea. We kept replenishing his cabin daily. He worked closely with assistants, and never asked where the supplies came from, probably being in no doubt. By the end of the voyage when we discreetly moved back to the signallers the crates were nearly empty.

Cape Town was living up to its postcards, with the table cloth thickly spread on the mountain. The other New Zealand transport, the *Ulimaroa*, had preceded us by two days and was tied up alongside an Australian transport. All the troops, over one thousand, combined for a Church parade on the Sunday, marching behind a band, ship by ship down the main street. The parade was led by the senior officer available who happened to be our Medical Officer. It was probably his first march and was quite creditable except that, according to the band, he was out of step the whole way. After the head of the columns had filled the first church, the residue was marched on to the second . . . and the third. It was a gaily ecumenical method and as such completely apartheid-free. The service I sat through was, I think, Methodist, though it was hard to tell.

John Nagle and I went to Camps Bay and up to the Groote Schuur, where we paid a toll of half a crown each to an elderly Negro. That evening, so we heard, he was back in gaol for illegally collecting tolls. We explored the beautiful gardens, and I remember still the wide clean gravel paths, the trailing blue wistaria and in the art gallery, a magnificent portrait by Franz Hals.

Three thousand miles of warming days and sometimes oily seas, phosphorescent trails at night and then the anchor dropped in the great harbour at Sierra Leone. Here for a dreary week Freetown was a bluish smoky ridge far across the slow currents of the wide muddy estuary. In the harbour were many vessels, some emptied by the influenza pandemic. On shore there were one hundred deaths a day, said those who had no means of knowing any figures. There were no cases on our transport for no one embarked or disembarked. This was in contrast to the *Tahiti* which followed us with the 40th reinforcements where the mortality at Freetown earned it the name of 'the death ship'.

We were visited by many canoes full of natives, dark, active, scantily clad little men. Some had a small English vocabulary, learned, so they said, at a missionary school. They made signs that they were hungry and were tossed some loaves of stale bread. They dived after them, squeezed the water out and wolfed the bread. In similar fashion they ate dubbin sandwiches. When the bread ran out they became abusive and the troops pelted them with potatoes from some sacks on deck. Most of these were either caught or rescued by diving. When the potatoes were exhausted and some canoes were full they paddled off to the shore, waving gaily. It was obvious we had underestimated their intelligence.

After a miserable week of flat monotony one evening the harbour suddenly filled with vessels. In the morning we could count forty destroyers as well as troopships, tankers and liners. At dusk that evening a heavily armed cruiser, an obvious flagship, moved out and the *Tofua* fell in behind. The convoy followed. At sea we all had our defined positions and kept them. We saw no more of the Japanese cruiser that had escorted us from Australia. The destroyers darted in and out of the convoy like fox terriers.

We were entering the war zone. Our naval gun behind the hospital was manned night and day and members of the medical corps were often detailed as ammunition guards. There was the strictest of blackouts. At night we probably went at half-speed, for an old grain-carrying tramp in the convoy which was out of sight every evening was leading the convoy the next morning. Each ship at night trailed a large brown barrel and the following ship rode on it. During the day armed sentries were posted on all ships fore and aft, port and starboard, scanning the sea for torpedoes.

John Nagle and I were leaning over the rail. The morning sick parade was over. The destroyers weaved in and out, cutting across our bows, racing to the horizon and racing back. Suddenly, one well out to our port bow fired one of its guns. Far astern a column of spray rose. Almost immediately another shell from another vessel landed near by. The alarm went and we ran to our stations. A destroyer at full speed shut us away with an impenetrable screen of black smoke. Shortly the All Clear was sounded. A submarine had been sunk, said our friends the Divisional Signallers.

That afternoon, again at the rail, we watched curiously a turmoil in the sea about two hundred yards away. The water was surging as if with the force of a subterranean spring. One of us idly suggested it might be a submarine. But it was not our discovery. A destroyer in close proximity sent two shells in rapid sequence into the turbulence. The alarm sounded throughout the convoy. Standing by our rafts (no boats) we could not see the end of the drama. When the All Clear sounded the sea was calm, the convoy unbroken and far astern two destroyers were moving in small circles. That evening two vessels which had been appearing and disappearing all day on the horizon came back together, flashing signals. 'Another submarine sunk,' announced our signallers.

'That's three in one day,' said John Nagle. (They were the only ones on the voyage.) 'I don't like it. We're going to the war. It has no right to come to us.'

'It shows the enemy is getting frightened of our arrival.'

'So am I,' said John.

And the last port was London. In the English Channel the whole convoy disappeared one night and the little *Tofua*, unescorted, chugged up towards Southend. Our ten weeks' voyage was ending. Before us were the incredibly green and placid fields of England and forty miles away were the guns in France.

John Nagle and I for the last time were leaning over the rail. The ship was cold and deserted. It was tied up at the King George Vth docks after a fascinating day of sailing up the Thames. The infantry had disembarked for Sling Camp. An hour later the Signallers had followed. There remained only thirteen medical Other Ranks, to be called for at any moment. John was pensive, moody and silent. I said little. Now I was in London. The occasion was too vast for chatter. A year ago, on the far edge of the world, I had been a serf in a minor protectorate of cows and turnips. This was my mother's home. A light fog clouded all but the immediate buildings. I would find it hard to believe I was here till London convinced me with some tangible proofs.

Suddenly John said, 'It looks bigger in the fog.'

'What does?'

He jerked his thumb above some rooftops. Here was only fog, though in the fog was a darker curved shape.

'What is it?' I asked. He rounded on me. 'Wake up, you damn fool. It's the dome of St Paul's.'

Ewshott was a dingy barren sort of camp, a mere scatter of huts. Gladly we left it for ten days' draft leave. The camp staff did their best for us: accumulated pay – paymaster; 'Never risk venereal disease' – padre; 'Never get venereal disease' – Medical Officer, supervising the compulsory issue of four condoms and two tubes of mercury ointment per man; leave pass and free railway tickets to furthest relative – Adjutant. The furthest relative was always in Inverness and my ticket was so endorsed without my knowledge. My only relative in the British Isles was possibly my grandfather Harrow's sister. He suspected her death as she had ceased writing. I found the address. The wispy fragile old lady who opened the door a crack bore an unmistakable resemblance to her brother. She was less sure of me. I had to explain my place in the family from several angles before she would let me in. She was still mistrustful. She made a cup of weak tea and a wafer of bread and butter. She asked how far I had come and again I lost ground. No two places could be so far apart as twelve thousand miles. I left with her about two pounds of precious sugar. (The quartermaster on the ship had urged us to indent heavily for sugar and fill our kitbags. Otherwise, owing to some quixotry of international tariffs and customs it would all be dumped in some harbour.) I thought the gift would at least bring a smile to that weary old face. Instead all her suspicions returned. Only a thief would have that much sugar and only a fool would so dispose of it. We parted, I am sure with mutual relief. Poor old soul, dying in the loneliness of London and with no relatives except an eccentric brother in a far land who had sent his mad grandson to spy on her.

Leave in London for O/Rs invariably meant booking in at the Shakespeare Hut in Bloomsbury Square. From here I did the traditional sallies into London: St Paul's, Westminster, the Embankment, Big Ben, Piccadilly. I went on my own, John Nagle having gone straight to his parents in Leeds. After a couple of days I received a telegram inviting me to join him. I would willingly have done so but my pass was to Inverness and Leeds was on another line. So I set out to get the ticket changed but could find no appropriate authority. Defeat followed defeat, perhaps the most humiliating being when I marched into what turned out to be a club for retired generals and admirals. Eventually I found a hearty New Zealand sergeant who came from some bush obscurity in the King Country and who was now an authority on London. He was in charge of some stores and had maximal leisure. I laid my problem before him. Had he any advice? He certainly had. To hell with Leeds. Go to Brighton. He was going to Brighton in a couple of days. Beautiful girls in Brighton. He had more than he could handle . . . . I persuaded him at last that my preference for Leeds was personal and not pleasure, and the only advice I wanted was where to get the ticket changed. He looked at me incredulously, then reached for my pass. He slapped it up against a brick wall and, after licking the stub of a pencil he ruled out Inverness and wrote above it 'Leeds'. And on this I travelled without question.

Two days in Leeds among kindly gentle folk who could not do enough for a friend of their John. I was taken through some of the steel works and munition works. They gave me genuine Yorkshire pudding and I gave them sugar.

On the notice board back at the Shakespeare Hut were details of a soldiers' excursion to Stratford-on-Avon the next day. To me it was more a pilgrimage than an excursion. At Stratford we were taken in charge by an elderly white-haired Shakespearean scholar who was more interested in the poet than in the sights. He could well be imagined as a retired University man who in the restrictions of war, was doing what he could with his talents. He obviously expected no high academic standard in colonial troops, but he served them well, putting himself pleasantly at their service. At the same time he was a subtle examiner, studying our faces, asking questions, probing for those who knew some Shakespeare.

Several did but no one else in our little group of a dozen had sat under Mr Rockel in the fourth form. My interest must have been obvious. At his request I finished some of his quotations. Thereafter I became his protégé. He took me into another room and showed me some precious folios but though I was a Shakespeare enthusiast I was no Shakespeare scholar and understood little of this.

Later, we were in the room where Shakespeare was born. I was examining the famous window with its many signatures. Our guide invited me to add mine and handed me a diamond stylus. I found a corner and wrote. I noticed that a nearby name was that of Walter Scott.

At the time I thought little of it – a signature such as might go in an autograph book. But the mystery of how it got there has deepened with time and greater knowledge. It is an honour usually reserved for the famous, the only qualification being merit. Perhaps my guide was indulging an egalitarian whim. Perhaps I was signing in honour of my country, for the news had just come through that the New Zealanders had captured the walled town of Le Quesnoy. (I learned later that the assault up the ladder had been led by Lieutenant L. C. L. Averill of whom I had never heard but who was to be a colleague for fifty years.) But, motives aside, the signature was made and is still there as a recent investigation (and photo) has verified.

That exciting day should have finished when I arrived back in late evening at the Shakespeare Hut. But I discovered with alarm that I had not booked one of the trestle beds in the large dormitory. Here we slept more soundly than securely with our uniform under the mattress, the money belt strapped round the waist and the top legs of the bed in our boots. I waited with other homeless ones till two trucks (Red Cross or Salvation Army or Y.M.C.A.) arrived and we filled them up. They shed their passengers in twos and threes at various hostels and moved off again immediately. I accordingly found myself in a dingy, stale-smelling hotel, part of a queue slowly moving up to a wiremeshed window which was presided over by an aged, irascible, uniformed lieutenant-colonel. Over his counter was a notice that no accommodation would be granted to anyone who had not been in France. 'All paybooks must be presented.' I decided to talk my way past this regulation but just then the colonel began shouting at someone in a like predicament. He knew his stuff, that colonel. He had been given a very minor part in the war effort but he was going to discharge it punctiliously, in which I was not going to help him at the cost of personal humiliation. I left the queue at one a.m. and went out in the dark streets of London, with a few coins in my pocket and a totally unjustifiable confidence in my sense of independence.

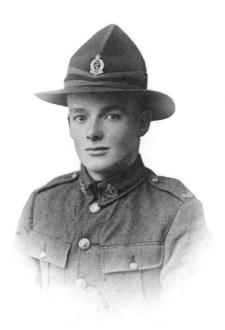

Private Bennett, London, 1918

I started walking in the vague direction of the Shakespeare Hut and was suddenly aware of my utter weariness. At first I passed a few pedestrians but none could help me. (How often are the pedestrians of London strangers to London.) But soon I was the only one in the deserted streets with great buildings on either side silhouetted against the inconstant sky as the clouds raced over the face of the moon.

What a fantastic city is London, hounding its millions through the sprawl of the day and draining all life from the night. I passed a large park with iron railings, then came residences, warehouses, shuttered shops, more houses and more shops, where old women with black shawls over their heads huddled in the corner of doorsteps. I hurried on. Their predicament was my predicament, that of no bed, but theirs alone was the tragedy. How cruel and indifferent London can be, despite its majesty. How inferior to Fairview in the matter of makeshift beds: no straw stacks, no mountains of pine needles, no hollows among the sacks of chaff. I decided I would go back to the park and look for a mattress of leaves under an oak, but the park had now vanished. From afar off the lilting strain of a dance band rode the night air.

Suddenly it was all very peaceful. Exhaustion and flat feet had halted me in a doorway. Then I saw someone approaching, a pedestrian on the other side, an early or late workman perhaps from whom I would force information. I crossed the street. As I confronted the other the moon suddenly lit us both and left me dismayed as I realized the other was a woman in a nightdress and slippers who had been sleep-walking and that I had woken her. She gazed at me with horror. Before I could explain she began to scream, piercing, reverberating screams, echoing and re-echoing over London. I fled literally doubling round corners in my first and only flight from a woman. It was not cowardice, merely a strategic retreat in the best military tradition. I would of course have been vindicated by the truth but even the truth might limp over the claim that a uniformed digger on the run and a scantily clad screaming woman represented only an accidental encounter.

The screams had stopped. Before me was a large solid looking hotel unlit and lifeless. It was no use knocking: I had tried this already this evening on a number of hotels, but no one would answer; yet now the need was greater.

A voice came out of the darkness:

'Looking for a bed, digger?' He stepped out of the shadows. He was a Y.M.C.A. padre from a country other than New Zealand. He was young, fresh-faced, sandy-haired, friendly.

'Well, I want a bed too. You wait here. I know this place.'

He disappeared up a side alley. A few minutes later he opened the front door.

'I've got a room,' he announced, handing me one of two lighted candles. We went up three flights of a creaking staircase. The bedroom was large and shabby with a double bed in the centre and a single one by the wall. He invited me to take the double bed. I, being a private, insisted that he have it. He then wanted me to have it with him. Warmer, he said. I wasn't cold, I assured him, and fell into the single bed and slept. A few minutes later I awoke to find him trying to get into my bed. I objected. He persisted. I suddenly became angry. I shoved him off and threatened that if he came back I would knock him out. He retreated, muttering:

'You don't understand, digger. There's a lot you don't understand.'

He was right. I did not understand the nature of his malady. I had encountered it in novels and vaguely in Shakespeare where it was displayed in taut academic dress, and was never clearly understood. I was asleep again before he got back to his own bed. There were no more interruptions – as far as I knew. In the morning I was up and dressed before he woke. I tried to force on him four and sixpence which was my share of the accommodation. He would not have it. We must meet again. He knew London; he would show me about. He would like to discuss certain things with me. He was busy this morning but could we meet for lunch? Say Piccadilly at twelve noon. I agreed but insisted that if he were not strictly on time I would not wait. He readily agreed. He would be there.

He was not. I gave him two minutes and thirty seconds, and then departed swiftly. He had possibly lined up a more suitable hotel partner for that night. I did not like him. I also do not like the fact that I still owe him four and six.

Back to camp. There were brave tales of adventures, some of them probably true, an interesting list of venereal casualties, and some surprising AWOLs. The first man back was one who could not read or write and was exiled by the written word. The ticket in his hand told him nothing. The name of the station had no meaning. After five exhausting days he was led back to camp.

A minor ordeal of the military life was surprise kit inspections. The soldiers resented this partly because it indicated suspicion and partly because the suspicion might be verified. For instance on the *Tofua* one of our more saintly conscientious objectors had protested strongly against having to empty his kitbag, which was found to contain five tunics and eleven pairs of slacks. There was a surprise kit inspection the day after our return. All our standard issue was stacked in the prescribed order and on top were our private personal possessions. Prominent among my modest assets was a copy of *Notre Dame*. It was an impressive volume in white hard-boards with gold lettering. The inspecting officer usually picked it up, spilled its pages beneath his thumb, changed it for a dingy copy of *Religio Medici* alongside, put them down, looked at me curiously, and passed on. But on this occasion the officer lingered. When had I learned my French? How long at High School? Did I take French? Was I the medical student? He passed on.

The next day I was summoned by the Adjutant who wanted me to confirm my French qualifications. Then he picked up a French newspaper. 'Translate this,' with his finger on a column.

Journalistic French is always easy. I had not gone far when he stopped me.

'Right. Now we want you for the N.Z.E.F. Educational Scheme Instructor in French. Run it your own way. Stationed in Ewshott at present. Rank of warrant officer, pay of a private. All right?'

'No sir.'

He looked up sharply, 'And why?'

'I would greatly prefer action in the field sir. I have never been to France and men who have spent years there would resent my trying to teach them.'

'Then we'll get someone else. You won't be asked again. You're a damn young fool. Get back to your unit.'

The Educational Scheme, of which more later, must have come from the fevered brain of some crazed educationalist. The syllabus seemed to include any subject for which a teacher could be found. The instructors were to be noted more for their personal courage than for their suitability. For the O/Rs (and possibly for the officers) two lectures a week were compulsory. Take your choice but there had to be two. I put my name down at Ewshott for a course in philosophy. At the first meeting the only other member of the class was a spidery little Scot who was determined to appropriate all he could from the army, and so went to a lecture every night of the week with bland indifference as to the subject. Our lecturer appeared. He was a solid middle-aged warrant officer. He said, with his eyes on the floor, 'My subject tonight is pragmatism'. We settled to listen. It sounded interesting. It could have been a disease or some cultural system from Prague or even a racehorse. But, though we listened for an hour to his monotonous dreary words, his eyes all the time fixed a yard or two in front of his boots, we had no idea at the end what pragmatism was. Thereupon I changed my course as I had a right to do. Nothing mattered as long as I went to two lectures a week.

We were retained in Ewshott for one purpose only: to learn gas drill. All the hours of training every day we carried gasmasks and much of every day we wore them. A gasmask is a clumsy device: a bag fitting closely over the face and forehead with nasal clips to prevent nasal breathing, connected by a tube to a cannister on the chest. Though clumsy it had of course to be reduced to a drill. A British drill sergeant could produce a drill for going to bed or being seasick. But we could not do gas drill for eight hours every day and in the intervals we marched in England's green and pleasant land. It was incredibly green in the depth of winter and as tidy as if it had been done over for a thousand years. We had to acknowledge a new agricultural standard. We might have fences and paddocks but in Hants they had hedgerows and fields. We had shelter breaks of pine. They had the lonely imperturbable oaks.

Then one day we were marched the four miles to Aldershott for our final examination in gas drill. We were warned that the examining sergeant had no natural love for colonial troops, especially for such as us, mere tyros in gasmanship. He shouted and barked and we dutifully popped in and out of gasmasks. But one of our number, terrified of the front line, made a bold bid for rejection by putting his fingers inside his gasmask to clean the eyepieces. The mask of course should have been invaginated from the outside. The enormity of the offence reduced the sergeant to a state of shock. He pointed at the culprit with a shaking finger and in a weak voice kept repeating, 'Oh my gawd, look what he's a-doing of, look what he's a-doing of'.

We never knew the sequel. He was removed then and there from our ranks and we never saw him again. Probably shot after dark by the sergeant as a matter of conscience.

The last item of the day was to convince the perverse diggers that the masks were effective. We marched through a closed dugout in the side of a hill. It was full of tear gas and we wore masks. We lingered long enough for a few breaths and then marched out. We had been unaware of any gas. Then we piled our masks and went through again. The first door slammed behind us. When we began yelling to open the other door the sergeant couldn't find the key and then discovered that he had not got it. Some of us by this time were in distress. We attempted to break down the façade of the dugout. Eventually someone outside was alerted by the noise and at last the door was opened and we tumbled out. Many of us were in a bad way but I was the worst of all. I lay on the grass strip opposite the dugout for nearly half an hour, struggling to get adequate air into my lungs. When I recovered and was able to take deep and glorious breaths, our camp Medical Officer questioned me about previous attacks. Then he said, 'I think we'll have to board you. The front line's too tough for you.' At once I protested. I was now all right. It had never happened before, it would never happen again. It was the old flat feet argument, losing nothing in persuasiveness because the language now had to be more discreet. He offered me a ride back to Ewshott in a truck. I insisted on marching.

Two days later there appeared in routine orders the names of six men who were being transferred to France the following evening. Mine was among them. John Nagle was not. We spent the next day in and out of the orderly room and in general preparations. We marched to Fleet Station and were in our train by six p.m. It was scheduled to leave in five minutes. But at six thirty it was still there. Then a corporal came galloping from camp and pulled us out. 'Back to camp,' he ordered. 'Rumours of an armistice. All reinforcements stopped.'

All reinforcements stopped. A year of effort and twelve thousand miles, all negated by twenty five miserable crawling minutes. Was it worth it? A good soldier goes where he is sent. All reinforcements stopped.

What now? There were four New Zealand transit camps in Torquay where embarkation drafts were assembled. Number Four Camp in an old English mansion was the hospital for them all. Here I became a hospital orderly, which might have pleased some people but did not please me. How many hospital orderlies have won the V.C.? In the hospital there were a few nurses, a new and pleasant association despite their habit of issuing orders: the lifting and carrying of wash basins and bed-pans, medicines and temperature charts, mealtrays and dressings; or anything else if the matron's eye happened to linger on you for a moment. Yet in the eyes of the world it was active service, which made it seem a little better.

The armistice was no surprise to Torquay, but its citizens preferred to treat it as such. The day was cold and misty and the traffic minimal. Suddenly, in mid-morning afar off, a siren sounded and a chorus of sirens answered. As they died there could be heard the measured dignity of bells. But they were swamped in turn by a hollow boom of sound. Below the hospital two men blowing cornets marched out of a side street, wheeled right and went down the hill. People with drums, whistles and mouth-organs poured out of the houses and fell in behind them. They were on their way to the greatest carnival of rejoicing in the history of man.

A military camp immediately lost all meaning. Camps were the outposts of war and there was now no war. It was a day for soldier and civilian, victors both, to dance in the streets. And only one voice was raised in opposition. There was to be no leave, said the Camp Commandant, no leave for anyone. Poor silly old man. He apparently thought that those whom the enemy could not stop in Europe or the Middle East could be stopped by him at the wrought iron gates of an old Torquay mansion. Some of the Anzacs from Gallipoli were in the camp. Their index of submissiveness was low.

The men dressed as for leave and marched in a body to the camp gates. The two guards while putting up a token resistance were lifted shoulder high and headed the jubilations rolling down the hill. Thereafter, all day, the gates stood open.

At the bottom of the hill digger met digger from the other camps and they all set out to capture Torquay. This they did as soundly as they had captured Le Quesnoy. The first attack was on the bars. Any barman who demurred at dispensing free beer, was relieved of his duties by someone who had probably trained in the King Country or in Hokonui. Such men were gentle, generous and persuasive. They welcomed civilians and responded to civilian tastes. The streets rapidly filled with noisy stumbling people.

Before long dancing (which requires balance) had to be abandoned. In the centre of the city, at the foot of the hill where the tramlines met, a group of diggers sat on the rails the whole afternoon playing two-up. Whenever one was dragged away another crawled into his place.

Finally the tramwaymen abandoned their trams and joined the throng on the pavement. One man high up a monument was orating against the noise. He was telling the people of Devon how Bill Massey had won the war. An old woman, very drunk and very down-at-heel blundered into me and stumbled on. I heard her mutter, 'Peace, perfect peace', referring I presume to her mood rather than to the international situation. Up the hill came a lanky digger with a newspaper full of fish and chips, punctiliously donating one chip to everyone he met. An hour later I listened again to the man who was still up the monument. His views had changed. New Zealand had now won the war despite Bill Massey.

There is no satisfactory formula for public rejoicing. Dancing, singing, spectacles of prowess or pageantry, processions, oratory, religious services . . . they are all outer garments covering the compass of goodwill and benevolence. So it was in Torquay. The crowds roamed the streets, soldier and civilian, male and female, arms linked, laughing, shouting, going nowhere, seeking nothing except the present, all cares lost on the way, all ages back to the irresponsibility of youth. *Gaudeamus igitur*.

A lovely country is Devon, profuse in its scenery and its interest. I did solo route marches on the frosty roads towards Newton Abbott, went to Plymouth to see the All Blacks draw with the Royal Naval Depot, played for the camp against the same naval depot the next week at Torquay where we repeated the draw. A mate and I took two Sisters for a day's sightseeing on the river Dart. This association of officers and O/Rs was of course unpardonable by English standards. But we were more interested in English scenery and English history than in English mores. And we had a grand day.

We had generous hours off duty except when overtime was necessary in a full hospital. One such occasion was during the great influenza epidemic of 1918. The hospital was crammed with patients who usually had a week of discomfort and then were returned to their units. A few (I would think not more than six) incurred a secondary pneumonia and died. We could do nothing for them except methodically administer some expectorant. The pulse and temperature were meticulously recorded even when the patient was grey, unconscious and panting. It was rather like polishing the brass on a sinking ship. The mortality was only a fraction of what occurred in New Zealand and this in turn was much less than we were led to believe through our N.Z.E.F. news sheet. (All my mail from home stopped about this time. A few months later in New Zealand I received forty-two letters on one day.)

I took a correspondence course in Pelmanism where I had to swear a mighty oath that I would not divulge the secret basis of the system. As it was never clear what was the secret method there was never any anxiety over the oath. It showed a slick method of remembering a list of related headings, but for an examination where the items were unrelated it was useless. I also took a course in shorthand and gained a certificate of proficiency. It was the Sloan-Duployan system, now as defunct as my memory of it.

Another unfortunate effort was derived from the ship's magazine on the *Tofua*. I had won a poetry prize and the editor asked me to write again for the second issue. This I did, but the second issue was never published. These verses I then sent to *Chambers Journal* in Edinburgh which published them and completely unbalanced me by submitting proofs, referring to my 'esteemed contribution' and paying me ten shillings and sixpence, which, in case anyone is now inclined to sniff, was nearly a week's pay. The consequences were wholly bad. I thought I was a poet and in the Y.M.C.A. hut attached to the hospital I wrote (and subsequently burnt) many pages of pointless rhymes.

I became the permanent locum at our hospital. I did overtime for other people and took the duties of those who wanted weekend leave. Every such duty was reported to the Sergeant-Major who assured me that it would be added to my annual leave. My intention was to tour the Lake District in the steps of the Lake poets. 'You've made a note of it, Sergeant-Major?' 'Yes, I've made a note.'

In the Torquay camps were now many of the original Anzacs for they were being repatriated in the order of their arrival. This meant that I would have to wait about a year. Then I heard of some New Zealand troops who were living in camp on army pay and going daily to London University College. This was a situation utterly desirable. I prepared my application with great care weighing every word. I opted for an Arts course and thought it safe enough to reveal that I had once been a medical student.

It was a calamitous letter. Two days later I was on the next embarkation draft leaving for New Zealand in less than a week. I went to the Adjutant. No, he could do nothing about it. I went to the Sergeant: 'What about that leave I was promised?' 'Yes – well we'll have to look into that.' 'But I'm leaving on Thursday.' 'We can always write to you.' 'You can't send leave in an envelope. Get me off that embarkation list.' 'Look, digger, you're bloody lucky to be on it. As a friend I wouldn't do anything to shift you.'

We left Torquay on a grey misty afternoon, shrinking in our greatcoats in the unheated carriage of the troop train. There was no meal before we left and no provision for food on our night-long journey to Liverpool. But – so we were told – the train would stop at Bristol where there was a large restaurant. There would be plenty of food, provided we had the money.

Before midnight the train stopped. The restaurant was large and ablaze with light. We poured out and raced towards it. A woman, just inside, yelled to someone behind her:

'Look out, they're New Zealanders.' She reached the doors before we did and slammed and locked them. A man came running and barred the companion doors. The lights went out. We yelled and hammered and there was talk of getting a jemmy. But some officers appeared and some M.P.s sauntered up. We got back and were hauled out in the darkness again. At least the exertion had raised the temperature a fraction.

Some of the men seemed confident that we would get generous leave in Liverpool. The train crawled down the wharf in the grey dawn. Our carriage door opened and we stepped down on to the lowest rung of a gangway up which we marched with an armed guard on either side. The train then moved on the length of a carriage and the process was repeated. England left us in no doubt that our services and our presence were no longer required. And the next morning we were out on the turbulent Atlantic with ominous weather coming up.

The *Athenic* soon declared its purpose which was to transport the largest number of bodies in the shortest time from Liverpool to Wellington. The circumstances were favourable. It was a fast ship, there was only one port of call and there was no tacking, no submarines, no convoys and no half-speeds at night.

My cabin, previously a hold, was occupied by four hundred and seventy-nine others. The hammocks were slung too closely together and the last man in each row was dispossessed. This meant that for a few nights I slept in a corner of the hold. There was some advantage in this for just below the hammocks were the mess tables and it was disconcerting when one's morning porridge had to be moved hastily to avoid contact with the bare foot of a late riser.

There was a number of soldiers' wives on board and a liberal sprinkling of babies. There was also a hospital to which the very seasick were moved early. Hearing of this I waited for the inevitable. 'We need help in the hospital,' said the Medical Officer. 'I believe you've had hospital experience and that you're a medical student.' There was a cubby hole near the hospital where my minor frame might rest at night. 'By all means,' said the M.O. when I put it to him. So I brought my kitbag and palliasse out of the hold. The hospital was similar to that at Torquay. The nursing staff was minimal. Some women patients were admitted and I was excluded from them. But there were more babies than women. A seasick woman could stay in her bunk provided she was relieved of her baby which was admitted to hospital. I was first given some minor tasks in the infants' section and then the scope increased. It was the first time in my life I had met babies and they fascinated me. Their great large eyes were full of innocence and trust. Had I been Rasputin or Bluebeard they would have refused to believe it and would have firmly grasped my finger in complete confidence. It was these babies who made me think again about medicine. A year before I had aimed to be a machine gunner. Now, the same hand was holding a feeding bottle and I had to admit that the latter was the more worthy task. A Sister showed me how to deal with a baby's wind. Two of them, very amused, stood over me while I changed a nap. Let them laugh. It was a vital service to a helpless subject and no laughing matter.

By and large it was an unhappy voyage. The original Anzacs were great fighters and when the target was sealed off by the armistice the martial fires died slowly. Protest meetings (of which the officers knew nothing) were held in the large hold. It was incredible to me how some minor matter thrashed over emotionally could become a major issue. The greatest indignation followed a premature birth on board and the baby's committal to the deep 'without a Christian burial'. I made some enquiries of my M.O. and at the next meeting I informed them that the premature birth was a miscarriage of six weeks and that if it had been formally buried a suitable coffin would have been a cigarette tin. I was howled down for this. To be on the side of 'them' and at so young an age was deplorable. Most of their complaints were deferred till a more appropriate time. This was to be the arrival at Wellington. Reporters from *Truth* were to be invited on board, and all the injustices detailed. Publication would follow and the whole world would know of the infamy. It was a thoroughly satisfactory solution, the more so because nothing was ever heard of it again.

In the first week at sea we were harassed by a pitiless Atlantic gale and the O.C. Troops, working together. The latter seemed terrified of any stuffy atmosphere in the sleeping quarters. So his men spent all day on deck huddling miserably in their greatcoats behind various superstructures from the lash of the storm and the whip of the waves. Though I have since spent a long time at sea, no maritime memory is as vivid as the misery of that seemingly interminable week in the Atlantic.

At length, in fine weather and riding blue seas we came to Colon where the grass was green, the distant hills violet, the palms were black silhouettes against the sky and the white blocks of houses were thick on the slopes. All our faith in the natural order of things came back. We polished our buttons and our shoes. Then – 'No leave,' said the O.C. Troops, 'No leave for anyone'. This must rank as one of the great military blunders of the war. They were Anzacs, they were militant, they were no longer seasick but they were sick of the sea, and had gone over the top in France.

Now they went over the top in Colon, scrambling down ropes to a sympathetic barge. Some officers came rushing up shouting. The men fell back and drifted away. It was too tame a surrender to be trusted. The officers went to the other side of the ship and found a full barge about to push off. They came back to the scene of their first victory. The barge now crammed was halfway to the shore. Another barge was manoeuvring into its place. Two more were approaching. The officers went below. Later the ship tied up to a wharf and a gangway was let down with an armed guard of two at the bottom pathetically demanding leave passes. Before long they too disappeared. The battle of Colon had been magnificently won.

The main objects of a large number of these stormtroopers were alcohol, women and tropical fruit. All were available but only the fruit was of good quality. The alcohol was devastating. It had the faculty of turning a genial personality into a dangerous belligerent. Conflict with the natives was almost inevitable. The New Zealanders had some German revolvers, the natives had knives. There was a rumour that lives were lost on both sides. Certainly we had some stabbed men in hospital.

The canal had to be traversed in daylight and so the journey had to start eight hours before sunset. But the next morning half the men were still on shore and a picket was sent to collect them. The next day a picket was sent to collect the picket. I was in a picket on the fourth day and we roamed the streets like a Salvation Army band urging all khaki-clad sinners to reform and return to the fold. On the fifth morning we sailed. Before we reached the first lock a barge crowded with troops came after us and were transferred. Even so, there were absentees of whose final fate we knew nothing.

The canal itself, coloured and picturesque, was a delight. To me it was a surprise. I had once won a Navy League prize for an essay on the Panama Canal, my information having come from a book on the subject. The canal I imagined and the canal I saw could hardly have been more different.

But out in the Pacific the way was long and the morale was low. The padres laboured with games, books, discussion groups. There were deck sports of the cruder type: greasy poles, crawling through the soot under a tarpaulin pegged out on the deck with a hose playing on top. There was also a boxing ring where the officers gave five shillings to the winner of the first bout every day. This tempted me on one occasion to accept the challenge of a man who was superior to me in reach but not in weight. What I did not know was that he was some provincial middle-weight champion. The bout was stopped in the third round. I could no longer fight because I could no longer breathe. Down below in the hold flat on my back on a form I took two hours to recover with various officers looking in on me. I am afraid I was a poor medical student. It was in the army that I confronted for the first time flat feet, homosexuality, asthma and the tantrums of babies.

The Educational Scheme was relentlessly prosecuted. Each soldier had to submit to two lectures a week, on any approved subject provided they were given by an appointed lecturer. There were only two such lecturers on the *Athenic*. One dealt with some aspect of the classics but as he was ill most of the voyage nearly all the lecturing was done by his colleague whose subject was poultry-farming. The consequences were pathetic. He was a demure little man of middle age who, I have no doubt, was excellent with his chooks but he was no lecturer. He would discuss the pros and cons of white leghorns and in the next lecture, black wyandottes. Then he would go on to poultry mashes, lice in hens, brown eggs and white eggs, building his lecture out of a mass of erratic diversions.

Inevitably the Educational Scheme had its conscientious objectors. Every scheme in the army does. These were the ones whose education had reached full completion and who were not going to risk an overload. For them physical drill was substituted, which involved various kinds of balancing feats on a crowded and moving ship and was turned into a burlesque by its participants. Still, apparently some official conscience would be satisfied.

The main diversion was gambling: poker, two-up and the ever popular Crown and Anchor. Its proprietors were generally noisy and rapacious and, unfortunately, successful. The players lost heavily, scraped and borrowed and lost again. There was on board as a member of the crew, a fresh-faced cabin boy who should have been at school but who was at sea, for there he got paid and so could help his widowed mother. I saw him one day invest a half crown on the board. He lost. He was immediately urged to double it on the same square. 'Double or quits.' It would have to turn up sooner or later. Foolproof system. Couldn't lose. And foolproof it was if one had the resources of a millionaire. The poor kid had no chance. From being the most insignificant person on board he had suddenly become the centre of a group of brave soldiers, all sufficiently concerned with his welfare to offer quantities of advice. Soon he was desperately trying to recover what he had lost. The game was stopped while he went below and came up with sixteen pounds, the total of his savings. He lost. Everyone sympathized. He stumbled away with a set smile on his pathetic face. The proprietor called him back. 'You're game, lad. You'll go a long way – here, take this,' and he flicked over a one pound note. There were murmurs of admiration. 'Good hearted bloke, old Pete. Always treats you decent.' My impulse was to snatch Pete's paraphernalia and fling it overboard. But I could not ignore the risk that I might have been made to follow it.

We were going back to a country still recovering from the loss of nearly seven thousand lives in the influenza epidemic. The severity, it was said, was due to the low immunity in the unsalted population in New Zealand. But New Zealand troops overseas were just as unsalted and yet were relatively immune. The inference was that the virus in New Zealand was of much greater virulence. On board, a zinc sulphate spray room was installed and through this everyone had to pass. Its supervision became a medical responsibility, which in the opinion of our M.O. meant mine. At the door I would check off the patients on my list, let them in, shut the door and fill the room with the spray hissing out of the perforations in the pipe running round the wall. I stayed with them for the statutory time, then let them out, opened both doors for ventilation and began to assemble the next group. Near the end of this duty I went down with the worst attack of influenza I have ever had. The zinc sulphate prophylactic ('fumigation chambers') had been used during the epidemic in some of the cities of New Zealand. It was quite useless, as was the mixed catarrhal vaccine (MCV1 and MCV2) given to all troops.

Towards the end of the voyage I, like all the O/Rs had to appear before an Education Officer, a certain Captain Garfield Stewart. Had I passed the Sixth Standard? I said a little haughtily that I was an undergraduate. Just so, but had I passed the Sixth Standard? I owned up and he ticked it off on the form. I added for good measure that I was a medical student. He remained impassive. Obviously he did not know what I was talking about. That same day I saw an O/R named Steenson flick a toffee paper at a tall lieutenant named Sinclair. It hit the latter on the cheek and he turned and growled 'Cut it out, digger,' to which Steenson replied, 'Oh shut up, you long slab'. The explosion I expected did not come. The officer, leaning on the rail went on moodily gazing at the ocean. A fortnight later Stewart, Sinclair and Steenson were all back at the medical school in their second year. (Stewart, a later firm friend of mine, did general practice for many years in Auckland; Steenson became a prominent medical officer in the Pacific, and Sinclair was killed on Mt. Egmont in mid-career.)

I dreaded the end of the voyage for though I had definitely decided to abandon medicine I had not only to tell my parents but to convince them. This was the difficult part for the reasons were not clear even to myself. Something deterred me from the study of medicine. I did not know what. But I persuaded myself that the real reason was financial. Board at Knox was one pound a week. Clothing, books, travel would absorb one

103

hundred pounds a year. Against this I had my deferred pay (actually I never saw it: my father said the vouchers came in very handy) and a trifle of a gratuity. Even though I worked all the holidays on the farm the main burden would fall on my father. His health was poor. My mother was trying to persuade him to sell the farm. If he did, his future would be austere. The Welfare State was twenty years away. No; no medical course. And the more I assured myself of this the more I regretted having to do so.

One morning a shout sent a rush of troops forward. There was a blue smudge on the horizon and as the day waxed it became part of a coastline and then, with surprising suddenness, part of Wellington harbour, and that evening we anchored somewhere off Massey Point. Here, for reasons to do with quarantine, we stayed for over twenty-four hours.

Wellington, dimly visible, was small and unpretentious, a straggling little place. It was a trivial apology for the great cities. In that miserable day of waiting I strengthened my resolution not only to abandon medicine but, before long, to abandon New Zealand. All the glamour and adventure was waiting across the sea. In Wellington the next day, idling time away in loneliness, I saw a middle-aged man bustling up some steps carrying a small bag. He was probably a householder whose wife had sent him shopping but it suited me to picture him as a doctor bent on an errand of mercy. Lucky man. How enviable was his state. All my doubts returned. If only I had some access to some money. The doubts travelled with me as the train rattled down through the parched Rakaia-Rangitata country. I lost them in a moment when I saw my father on the Timaru station. He seemed older, he was more bent. I should be supporting him.

The real family reunion was that evening. I had driven the car home with a Patriotic Society Union Jack flying at each corner of the windscreen, and strangers in the streets had waved and my father had waved back, but not till the evening was there leisure.

We sat round the green plush-covered table in the yellow circle of the kerosene lamp, with my brothers silent in the big shadows. I had brought little presents. My mother was wearing the lace shawl I had bought in Colon. We talked quietly, letting the conversation drift where it would. They told me of the news of the district, all the trivia of their neighbours. I answered their many questions. When a reference was made to my returning to the medical school I said nothing. I brought out my postcards, including all I could purchase of Woodgreen, none of which my mother could recognize.

At an hour which was late for them I saw my mother nod at my father and he said:

'There's something we have to tell you.'

He then told it, slowly and in detail as was his habit. It began with the newspaper notice, the interviews back and forth, the agony over the application form, the testimonials . . . .

'He did it all himself,' interrupted my mother proudly.

And then the finish. I had been granted a Returned Soldier's Bursary of fifty pounds a year for five years for the purpose of completing my medical course.

Their faces were animated but it was the hands that I remember: my mother's white and misshapen, yet capable of adding a push to the willpower which enabled her to ply a needle, and my father's, rough, calloused and work-grimed. They were hands that never failed before the end of the task.

I could reply with nothing but thanks and suddenly I meant it. No more running away. Any course other than the obvious was now unthinkable. A good civilian, like a good soldier, goes where his destiny sends him. Two days later I was in Dunedin.

6

Elusive Qualification

I was back in Knox College, greeted by Professor Hewitson the Master, Miss Manson the Matron, and by many of my erstwhile contemporaries who looked at me uncertainly as if wondering where I had been over a long weekend. So I put up an R.S.A. badge but soon took it down. They were as common as greatcoats in the Octagon in July. I looked at my former classmates with some disquiet. They were approaching the First Professional and were bleary-eyed, distrait, jumpy, and had been persuaded that the proper study of mankind was Anatomy. I suspected the medical course might have problems.

Yet, though once again I started late, it was an easy two terms in which to dispose of the rest of the Medical Intermediate. Then began Anatomy and Physiology. After one term of human dissection I went home for the long vacation in serious doubt as to whether I could go back. This time it was not the subject but the environment of the large dissection room with its formalin reek, its cold metal-topped tables, its permeating essence of death despite the chatter of the class convinced me that I had not the temperament for Anatomy. This is a common reaction of students but it is usually replaced in a week or two by interest in the subject. I had no interest in the subject – at least, as outlined in the dissecting room. I preferred Anatomy from a different angle:

> She was a Phantom of delight
> When first she gleamed upon my sight;
> A lovely Apparition, sent
> To be a moment's ornament. . .

Sir Gordon Bell, Professor of Surgery at Otago, in his autobiography *Surgeon's Saga* (Wellington, Reed, 1968) represents dissection as an exacting procedure. He began with the area behind the knee (the popliteal space) and I cannot resist giving a description of what he found:

Here was an arrangement, a disposition, so orderly, so logical and so sensible. . . .
In short, as it seemed to me, here was the perfect introduction to dissecting-room anatomy . . . . At any rate it gave me a permanent liking for the subject . . . .

A permanent liking for the subject! Had I not known Professor Bell and his integrity I would not have believed him. Anatomy revolted me.

In the midst of this indecision John Nagle arrived, squeezing all he could out of his free pass. He stayed a few days with us and was his usual silly, likeable, extravagant self. But it was soon clear that the old alliance was broken. The army had been our catalyst. I tried in vain to interest him in farming procedures. He was uneasy at our way of life, at my mother's twisted frame, at grace before meals, at the necessity to discipline his language.

But we could still talk, he and I, confidentially as we had done so often. I told him of my dislike of Anatomy. As usual his judgement was direct.

'Bloody little coward you are. Scared of mice too, I suppose. Don't you want to be a quack and save millions of lives? You must have a touch of brain fever lad. Phlebitis probably. All this poetry stuff. Now you get back on parade. Don't go and spoil things after the way I've brought you up.'

I took him down to the station after three days and I think our parting was with mutual relief. Loyalty would always remain but friendship was more than loyalty and the purpose of friendship had been served.

I never saw him again.

Many years later in the course of a crowded afternoon he rang me from the Christchurch station. I had to identify myself by many questions before he would give his name. But his voice and its careful low slurring made both him and his condition unmistakeable. I arranged the evening at my place. But he did not arrive and I had no means of tracing him. He must now be long dead. But to me at least he still lingers in kindly memory.

I went back to the Medical School, put on the white coat, collected the suture needles, scalpel and forceps and made a determined attack on Anatomy. But I could not sustain the attack. The names of the muscles and nerves I had so carefully learned one day I had forgotten the next. I probably spent twice as long as other students with my notes in front of me and I probably measured only a quarter of that time in concentration.

Because my method of learning was the thoroughly bad one of prodigious feats of memory and minimal feats of comprehension I was often unsure in exams. In written papers this could be disguised to some extent. But in oral exams there had to be a rapid crossfire of question and answer. If I hesitated my uncertainty grew. The position was aggravated by certain personality clashes with one of the Anatomy staff. My ineffectiveness in oral exams grew to the stage where I have often known the right answer but owing to an obsessional doubt as to its accuracy I have been unable to reply. The condition exists among a few unfortunate students. The cure is to saturate oneself in the knowledge of the subject till the hesitancy is replaced by the boredom of conviction.

By the end of the year I realized that the tide was running against me. Physiology, which I had neglected, suddenly became as ominous as Anatomy. I switched desperately from one to the other, and did no good at either. I knew the inevitable as I approached the First Preliminary and for once I was right. I failed both subjects.

This was truly the end. I would have to face a dreadful interview at home and then I would be free. Suddenly this was opposed by a number of my friends in Dunedin. They were a formidable group: John Cairney, R. S. Aitken, Jack Hinton, J. A. D. Iverach, all of whom later attained professorial status. Leading them was the Master of the College, Professor Hewitson. He insisted that I continue. 'You have other qualities,' he said. He gave me faith in myself and reduced the mountain of Anatomy to a mere pebble in the path. He paid my fees for two terms at Knox.

So I continued, as by now I secretly wanted to. John Cairney, later to be associate professor of Anatomy and later still Director-General of Health, gave me a number of special coaching lessons, probably instigated and paid for by Professor Hewitson. He stressed only the important aspects. For the first time I began to see the subject from the examiner's point of view. A year later I sat the exam and passed. I pretended a nonchalance which was in deep conflict with the elation I felt.

There were new subjects: Bacteriology, Materia Medica and Pathology. They were interesting and could be mastered. I worked for a year and approached the Second Professional with confidence. But in that same week I developed a physical illness with cough and fleeting hallucinations. I sat the first paper and apparently doodled over several pages. The next day my chest was X-rayed (right chest densely mottled) and I was sent home by Professor Fitchett with a diagnosis of advanced tuberculosis and orders not to return till Dr Blackmore, Superintendent of the sanatorium, agreed. It was a miserable illness. I developed a peripheral neuritis and a bilateral foot drop and could not walk properly for about four months. The diagnosis has never been made. It was certainly not tuberculosis. Sarcoidosis has been suggested. Maybe. I spent my time at home which was now in Christchurch, the farm having been sold. I did household chores, wrote verse and articles for Christchurch papers, and read medicine. Dr Blackmore refused to see me. (He was feuding with Professor Fitchett at the time.) So I ordered myself back to Dunedin where Professor Fitchett was much surprised to see me. Shortly after, I passed the Second Professional.

This lugubrious tale of a poor student and a worse examinee would not be worth the telling if there had not been another side. I tried to respond to the cultural life of the University. I became junior and then senior secretary of the Medical Students' Association and a member of the Students' Council. I joined the Debating Club and also the S.C.M. (Student Christian Movement), ultimately becoming president. My winning entry in the annual literary society essay prize was on the art of Robert Bridges (there was a man who corrected me on my priorities: he became a doctor first and poet laureate second). I wrote for all the student publications and edited them in turn, with the exception of *Critic* and the capping magazine. One year I established a record which still stands and always will: to win the Macmillan Brown Prize for literature ('Tragedy is the highest form of literature' – a thesis I upheld then but would hesitate over now), to edit the University *Review* and to fail Anatomy. Anyone who attempts to break this record will need to repeat all of these events in the same year and this is not constitutionally possible.

The winner of the Macmillan Brown Prize automatically acquired a new status in the literary world of the undergraduates. This was particularly hard to assess in the case of an obscure medical student. But it was probably because of this that the Arts Faculty nominated me as Member for Intellectual Affairs on the Student Executive. A consequent duty was to edit the review. But my most pleasant memory is that, in effect, I founded *Critic*. My predecessor (Dan Aitken, my study mate) controlled a four-page publication known as *Te Korero*. It was a dismal rag which he and I usually filled up with imaginative froth a few hours before it went to press. When I succeeded him I moved at the annual meeting of the Old S.A. that *Te Korero* be replaced by a totally different production. The meeting agreed. I later presented detailed plans to the Executive and was told to go ahead. So *Critic* was born, with A. J. Campbell as editor and W. M. Searle as manager. Naturally it had teething troubles. Some students were critical. The cynics became eloquent. Many who approved refused to pay the two shillings annual subscription. The University authorities withheld their participation till respectability had been proved. I forget who suggested the title. It could have been me for it was certainly what I had in mind. Many years later I read that the editor had been sent down for a year. It was a splendid tribute to the virility of the periodical.

There were giants in the University in those days. The new student constitution which established the students' council of about seventy responsible members was the work of a law student, H. E. Barrowclough, later to be the general commanding the New Zealand Expeditionary Force in the Pacific, and later still Chief Justice of New Zealand. The first medical student to win a Rhodes Scholarship was Arthur Porritt, followed the next year by R. S. Aitken. Previously the medical student was regarded as boisterous, lacking graces, unaware of his poor culture. These two, each receiving a knighthood in mid-career, significantly shortened the bridge between medicine and the arts. There were others: Sir Douglas Robb, to be president of the B.M.A. both in England and New Zealand, and pioneer of cardiac surgery in New Zealand; Sir Charles Burns, physician of Wellington, a generous and indefatigable teacher; Sir Edward Sayers, later to be Dean of the Medical School; Sir Archibald McIndoe, plastic surgeon in Britain. At the student stage the future was hidden. Some became professors: Derek Dennis-Brown, Neurology, Harvard; Archibald Durward, Anatomy, Leeds; Eric d'Ath, Pathology, Otago; J. A. D. Iverach, Associate Professor, Medicine, Otago. There were some who were to be famous medical missionaries: A. Harvey, M. Ryburn, E. Sayers, A. L. Sutherland, Bramwell Cook and H. B. Turbott (later to be Director-General of Health).

One of the many advantages of living at Knox College was the association with and the friendship of those in other faculties. In my day there were Geoffrey Bellhouse, Alan Watson, and Mac Wilson, all to be Moderators of the Presbyterian Church respectively in Britain, Australia and New Zealand; Jimmy Salmond of church and college fame; Hubert Ryburn, a Rhodes Scholar and later Master of the College; Arnold Nordmeyer, destined for politics; Jack Hinton, demonstrator in Physics, who was to die tragically just after being appointed Professor of Physics at Colombo; Jimmy Leitch, president of the Students' Union, a staunch mining student from the West Coast, who also was to die tragically at an early age.

An outstanding personality even in student days was A. C. Aitken, later to be Professor of Mathematics at Edinburgh. My closest contact with him was at an S.C.M. conference at Geraldine. On New Year's Eve he demonstrated for us the mathematical wizardry for which he was famous. He squared huge numbers, found square roots without pausing, fixed a day to any date in the last century. He introduced us to the fraction 1/97 (or was it 1/93?). Converted to decimals it ran to ninety-three (or ninety-seven) places and then repeated. He knew them all and given any consecutive three figures could complete the rest. He it was who, when his platoon was shot up in France, was able to supply from memory the regimental numbers of all his men and the numbers of their rifles.

On that New Year's Eve in Geraldine there was more movement than Christianity. We marched through the one street with a sort of hill-billy band led by Aitken on his violin. He came round a corner and had a direct confrontation with the Temuka Pipe Band. We joined forces, discovered a vacant hall and announced an impromptu Hogmanay concert in honour of Geraldine. In twenty minutes the town, which had seemed uninhabited, filled the hall, children, dogs, Rip Van Winkles and all. The concert varied in its artistry, but socially it was magnificent. The pipes were very good and Aitken's parody of them on the violin was superb.

When the Scots deserted us, having secret midnight business elsewhere, we felt hungry. We found a small teashop, roused the owners (two elderly ladies) and ordered bacon and eggs for forty-five. After they had shown us their resources they were sent back to bed. The girls did the cooking, the men washed up and Aitken collected the money and left it under a plate on the kitchen table.

There were a number of visits by notable people. One was that of H.R.H. the Prince of Wales whose car swept down King Street past the Medical School and its gowned staff, and turned into the hospital, led by a medical students' 'band' with human bones simulating musical instruments. The Prince was more amused than was Dunedin. We were otherwise excluded from his hospital tour. This alone would have foiled the plan we had discussed of kidnapping him and taking him to Knox to play poker. The scheme was as impracticable as it was foolish. As he left we chased his car down Princes Street. He stood up in the back seat, turned round and watched us with amusement. As the car gathered speed and we had to give up, the leading man, now a professor of international fame, called, 'Hooray Teddy,' and the Prince waved back and called 'Hooray digger'.

Another famous visitor was Lord Rutherford. His address in the Physics lecture room was nominally to physicists. Almost the whole University staff was there. Presiding was Professor Jack, our erudite professor of Physics. All he and his visitor had in common was their subject. Lord Rutherford, burly, genial, untidily moustached, looked like a North Canterbury farmer who had just done well at the woolsale. Professor Jack, lean, jerky, anxious, looked as if his wool had arrived late and had been excluded.

Lord Rutherford spoke easily and casually and yet fluently. He amplified his introduction and referred to his physics laboratory. 'There is,' he said, 'only one Cavendish professor at Cambridge and . . .' he paused and then spread his hands in a gesture of deprecation, '. . . well, I am it.' He said that atomic physics tended to be a little complicated and he had no intention of inflicting it on his present audience. The principles, however, were simple enough. If for instance one took the formula . . . He spied a piece of chalk and wrote up a formula. He explained this with the help of two more formulae. By this time he was away. His address

111

resulted in a blackboard completely covered with symbols and equations. He turned away from the board as if to assure himself that his audience was still there. His favourite phrases were, 'It follows . . .', 'It is therefore obvious. . .', 'This results in. . .'. At the end the only man in the race was Professor Jack, sitting in the front seat, head cupped in hands, frowning at the board. We applauded the lecturer vigorously at the end. Anyone who could perplex Professor Jack in his own subject deserved it.

Other visitors in a minor key were the Oxford debaters, Woodruffe, Hollis and McDonald, the last being the son of Ramsay McDonald. My position on the Executive made me responsible for their day-to-day activities in Otago. Their debating was clever enough, but their subjects were so worn that some of the puns and epigrams had preceded them. They were not impressed by Knox nor by Otago University. I think their unresponsiveness, their eccentricities and their contempt for punctuality could only have been cultivated. McDonald alone seemed to respond to the Scottish atmosphere of Dunedin. As he left he invited me, if I ever went to London, to look him up. 'But don't jump in the first cab and say "10 Downing St." Make a few enquiries first.'

For a long period at Knox I sat next to D. G. McMillan, later to be a fierce critic of the B.M.A. in the first Labour Government. He was a lively conversationalist but none of us discussed politics. His earliest practice was at Kurow, where the tumbling waters of the Waitaki do not seem to encourage orthodoxy. Three rebels in the respective fields of politics, medicine and theology, A. H. Nordmeyer, D. G. McMillian and Lloyd Geering, all began their professional careers at Kurow.

The passing of the Second Professional effected a grand liberation. All the scientific background for which I was so ill-fitted had passed. Now came the clinical subjects, Medicine, Surgery and Gynaecology. Or in other words, men and women instead of test-tubes and microscope. Or in still other words, X-ray plates and temperature charts and stethoscopes sticking out of the pockets of long white coats. Behind was a long dark tunnel and in front were sunlit fields. For the first time, I ardently wanted to become a doctor. To a little group of friends, determined to purge me of vice, I had to swear that I would take no further part in any student activity, would do no writing and would campaign no more. The promise was kept.

But there remained Applied Anatomy. My emancipation from the dread subject was not yet complete. The night the results of the Second Professional were announced I got out Rawling's *Surface Markings* which is a primer in the subject of Applied Anatomy, and thereafter every single day for the next year I read, or thought, or mentally reviewed some aspect

Elusive Qualification

of the subject. And eventually all this was cashed in for a quite creditable pass in the exam.

The medical student of today faces totally different conditions. The syllabus has changed, the standard of Anatomy and Physiology fortunately has been lowered, the teaching staff includes many full-time professors, there is elaborate equipment and clinical material. The exam problem, of necessity, has to persist but it is not the sole arbiter of efficiency. All examiners recognize the student who is a poor examination subject. I was certainly one. After my failure in Anatomy I was appointed demonstrator to dental students in the dissection of the head and neck. Of necessity I had to learn the subject thoroughly, yet in the oral exam this subject gave me great trouble. (It is ironical that the first professional money I ever earned was for demonstrating Anatomy.) I once walked from Knox to the Medical School along with a class-mate who was appalled when I mentioned a likely question. He knew nothing of it except the name. Would I tell him something? I told him all I knew. The question was there. I got fifty-eight; he got sixty-four. The subject of Materia Medica was an appalling confusion of names, preparations and doses. It had no logic to it and I was certain I could never present it with confidence in an exam. If only it had been in verse . . . . So I took most of the difficult items and turned them into verse. It was crude and banal stuff but it had a swing, a rhythm and a rhyme and was therefore unforgettable. It served me well. In subsequent exams there was a little hesitation till I found the right disc to play, and after that, transformed into decent English, it flowed forth.

Dunedin Hospital could not of course supply enough clinical material. The first case of rheumatic fever I ever saw was presented to me for diagnosis and discussion in the final exam. The exception was at Seacliff mental asylum, where we went in small groups for a fortnight at a time. Here we were swamped with psychiatric patients. It was while there that I once saw a man, tall and erect with white beard to his chest and white hair to his shoulders. He was immaculately dressed in a white drill suit. He marched steadily down the corridor, eyes fixed on the distance, a startling figure, like a lost ancient prophet. This was Lionel Terry, the classic paranoiac who had shot and killed a Chinese to draw attention to his pamphlet on the 'Yellow Peril'. His mental disintegration at this stage was far advanced. Even ten years before, at the outbreak of war, he had attempted to cable to Sir Edward Grey. 'Stop all hostilities until I arrive – Terry.' Another patient was Matthews, the Timaru murderer, a gorilla of a man. With others, I was in his cell one day when he singled me out and suggested a couple of rounds with the gloves. I was polite but very firm.

113

He then wrote my name in an exercise book. A warder later informed me that I was now on the list of those marked for death as soon as he was free, but that there were over thirty ahead of me.

We owed much to our teachers who spared no effort to help. Some of the lecturers were general practitioners who must have worked a tortured time-table. They were all able teachers and some of them were very good. Only one, however, Professor Fitchett, could have been described as a born teacher. He appeared stern and humourless but this was a background for his brilliant wit. He was impeccably dressed and faultless in manner. By personality alone he ensured the attention of his class. He was a caustic critic and yet a kindly one. The verbal whip might crack at any time. ('And what are your grounds, Mr A, for assuming that this is your final year?') Alone of the lecturers he offered advice on general practice. ('Never neglect pregnancy as a possible diagnosis. Some women become pregnant if you merely pass them in a tramcar.') He warned against starting practice with too much hair on our heads and too little on our faces. In his teaching he favoured the dramatic. Describing his special treatment for acne he said, 'She was the worst case of acne I have ever seen. Her face was a revolting sea of pus. I applied the treatment. Did it work, you ask? Gentlemen, I have since confined her twice. Need I say more?' So that he became an inspiration to his generation and a legend later.

Of his teaching technique one example must suffice. We sat, the whole class, in the hospital amphitheatre. The young woman on the bed below had some red areas on her lower legs. He made us describe them, and then, turning to a student in the front row he said,

'Well now, Mr F – diagnosis?'

'I think it's Erythema nodosum, sir.'

'You think it's what?' incredulously.

'Erythema nodosum, sir,' uncertainly.

'Mr F, are you an authority on Erythema nodosum? Have you in fact ever seen a case?'

'No sir.'

'And yet you . . . .' He turned away wearily and appealed to the rest of us. 'Come now, what else could it be? Anyone? What else could it be?'

No one knew. Everyone tried, tried desperately, but no one knew. There were a few timid suggestions which he brushed aside. Finally he said:

'Well, let me tell you something, Mr F. If ever you should become a doctor and ultimately attract to yourself a few patients one of whom had lesions like these and you had the temerity to say it was a case of Erythema nodosum, at which all your colleagues laughed you to scorn, then my

114

advice to you, Mr F, would be to stick to your guns, because you would be right and they would be wrong. It is Erythema nodosum.' This was splendid teaching. No need thereafter to look up a picture in a book; not only had we seen the real thing, but despite ourselves had had it firmly fixed in a visual memory. The girl must be dead now but her lesson lingers – three spots on the left leg and two on the right.

The final year medical student, always excepting the brilliant ones who seemed to have inherited their knowledge genetically, usually approached the last exam as if he were the defendant on a charge of ignorance, and devoted himself almost exclusively to building up his defence. At Knox after chapel, which was unjustifiably compulsory on three evenings a week, and when a frequent hymn was 'Take from our souls the strain and stress', the College would be wrapped in silence till half past nine, when for half an hour there would be the racket of suppers as various groups acquired in turn their right to the kettle at the end of the corridor. Then silence until a new day would break to the boom of the gong parading the ground floor. (Overheard in the Opoho tram, one old lady to another 'Yes, that's Knox College. Terrible place. Those students. You'll see their lights going till after midnight. Playing cards the lot of them.')

In the last term there would be some short periods of furious application to tennis and fives, the rules of the game being secondary to the value of the exercise. In the interval between tea and chapel the golfers at one stage held a nightly putting competition at the back of the College, with the best scorer having the right to drive the ball of the worst into the tangle of the Woodhaugh gardens where many probably still are. One night, one student, later a staid practitioner of Ashburton, decided that the unbearable monotony of study should be broken. He therefore paid five shillings for a basket bomb, set it in a biscuit tin on the stone stairs of the College, and in the depth of a deep silence he engineered its explosion. It was said that the whole College shook for a few seconds. Certainly some students shook for a few days.

Halfway through the last term the clinical exams started. We were excluded from the hospital and each waited for the telephone call that was the summons to the new admission that had to be examined, diagnosed and treated. The air was thick with rumours. Everyone knew what was in the wards and everyone seemed to be wrong. False tips abounded and even the occasional correct one was still full of danger. (Professor Fitchett: 'Yes. Quite right. You should be proud to be the only person in the world who can diagnose optic atrophy in both eyes by examining one.')

Till, in the end, none of this mattered. We lost interest in the tricks. We lost interest in the last minute cramming. The more we sought clarity the more we found confusion. Faithfully we ticked off the items of papers, clinicals and orals in Medicine, Surgery, Obstetrics and Gynaecology.

There remained the epilogue. Early one evening we massed in the dingy common room of the Medical School. The last oral had been held that afternoon. The examiners had been in conference for hours. It was six o'clock and the bars were closing. There was a slow slur of conversation from little groups of twos and threes. It was disjointed, passionless and told of exhaustion.

Suddenly it stopped. Downstairs from the examiners' room came the year's representative (J. A. Paterson). He mounted the common room table and focussed the light on his list. To the blind there would have been nothing in that room but silence.

'The following have failed in all subjects.' It was a long list, a dreadful list.

'The following have failed in Medicine and Surgery . . . in Medicine, Obstetrics and Gynaecology . . . in Surgery, Obstetrics and Gynaecology . . . .' No sound competed with the flat voice, a mere conveyor of names.

'The following have failed in one subject only . . . .' And so on to the end.

Then the uproar broke. Doctor slapped doctor on the back and wrung the professional hand. It was as if the gates of the prison had been blasted away. It was all noise and shouting and there was no depth to it. The only depth was in the tragedy, for fifty percent of them did not cheer. They stood around, smiling bravely. There were unexpected additions to their ranks, and unexpected omissions. They left early in quiet groups, saying little, for each was planning the next term; new living quarters, new pattern of life, another term or year as a medical student, a new attack on the fortress of the final. The public do not know how vigilant on their behalf are the watch-dog examiners.

I had rented a house for a fortnight and had persuaded my parents to come down to the Exhibition. I rang my father and used my new title. He did not pick my voice and kept insisting that the owner of the house would not be back till the end of the month. Finally I had to spell it out for him. He said he was not surprised. What faith!

I went from the telephone to our old family Chevrolet which I had parked in front of the Medical School. It was already packed with doctors. The final total was nine. As we passed the Medical School the examiners in a body came to the top of the steps. The car rocked with our cheering and the horn added a fanfare. They waved back with the cordiality of colleagues. We went to the Exhibition which so far had been out of bounds. As a group, we got into the motor pavilion and were immediately

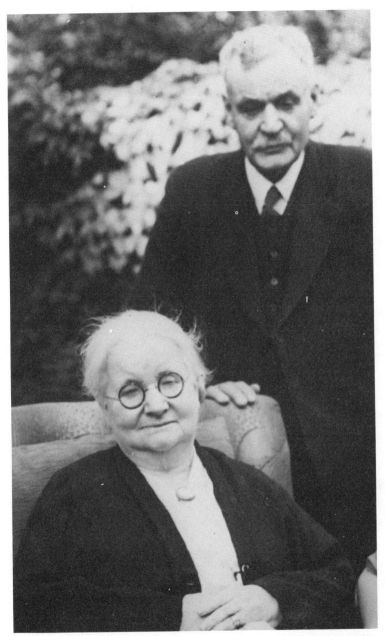

The author's parents, Rose and William Bennett, Christchurch, 1939

pinned down by ambitious salesmen who were more inclined to believe in our potential than in our insistence that we could not get home unless we hitch-hiked. The confrontation finished when we began buying an average of two cars each, signing forms usually with the names of film stars or politicians. In the end the salesmen massed and more or less rough-handled us out of their pavilion.

The next day I was back at the Exhibition, pushing my mother's wheelchair past show cases. We came on a display of fine needlework which had once (I think) belonged to Queen Victoria. I pushed at her command and our pace was about seventeen point six yards per hour. She was lost in the pageantry of the past; I was lost in the perfection of the future. It was a long time since I had worked the sewing machine for her but in effect our roles were still the same.

That night she began to write round the family to inform them that her son was a doctor. Poor mother! She never lost the silver lining to her clouds even when in later life she went blind. Even I knew (or was soon to learn) that I had hardly started to become a doctor, and if I was ever going to be a good one I would never cease to be a medical student.

The life of a medical student as here depicted refers to me only. Many doctors would render an entirely different account. I have no authority to speak for anyone else. Certainly many were happier in it than I was.

Neither of my parents had been in Dunedin before. We motored round a charming city, and kept going back to the Exhibition. It was a happy period. I packed my books at Knox (and still have some of them). We left after a fortnight; though the house was comfortable and fully-furnished it was costing four pounds a week. As we drove out up the valley, and past Knox, out of Dunedin, my parents were going back to their little home, and I was heading north to the great wide world.

7

Coercion on the Coal Face

For many reasons the newly qualified doctor should have a period as a house surgeon. But in the mid-twenties many medical superintendents discounted his worth and provided no vacancy. There were always more applicants than positions. Hopefully we all applied to the hospital of our choice before we sat the final. I was thus appointed to the Queen Mary Hospital at Rotorua, but the appointment was later overlooked and another doctor substituted. I learned of this while doing a locum for Dr Burns Watson of Lumsden. I wired urgently to Professor Hercus – a house surgeon's job, anywhere, any conditions. He received two other telegrams that day, one from a friend of mine who wanted a house surgeon's job, anywhere, any conditions; and another from New Plymouth Hospital where a patient had just died under an anaesthetic administered by a final-year student. 'Must be qualified,' added the wire. Professor Hercus differentiated between the two candidates by counting all their pass marks in all subjects in the previous two years. I won by one mark and a few days later was junior house surgeon at New Plymouth Hospital.

What did a house surgeon do in his day's work? I hardly knew but I was prepared to do it. I soon discovered that he did very little except for a twenty-four hour duty involving responsibility for new patients, minor surgery, assisting at operations, dressing wounds, giving anaesthetics, completing case notes, interviewing relatives, placating the disgruntled, writing death certificates, lecturing to nurses, doing day rounds and night rounds and infectious diseases rounds, explaining to Sister that it was all an oversight and will never happen again, making up the next day's diets for the diabetics, running an outpatient service without outpatient facilities; falling into bed at midnight and having a nightmare that the night Sister was knocking on the door because of a sudden crisis in Ward Two, and then waking to find it was not a nightmare after all.

The Superintendent was Dr Walker, a pleasant part-time surgeon who was on the point of retirement and who gladly left increasing responsibility to his house surgeons. The Assistant Surgeon was Dr

George Home of whom more will be said. On Dr Walker's retirement he was followed by the first full-time Superintendent, the late Mr J. M. Clarke of Auckland. The senior house surgeon was Dr Basil Wilson whose interests were surgical. Mine were medical. We made a good team.

It was a busy hospital. There was much traumatic surgery especially from accidents on Mt. Messenger, a high incidence of tuberculosis and a persistent prevalence of sick Maoris. Clinically, despite the bizarre and the unusual, the hospital was little different from any such hospitals throughout the country.

I remember the personalities better than the maladies. There was for instance the Matron, Miss Campbell, noted for her discipline of nurses, her office full of brass trophies, and her play with a fly-swat. She did not tap phones, but there was a number of instances where an outside phone got tangled with hers. Counter-measures resulted. For instance the Theatre Sister had to stay in most evenings in case of an acute operation. Despite this she was to be found on these same occasions at a certain house not far from the hospital, and if I rang this number and left a message that Jack would be arriving by car at seven p.m. on the nineteenth, the lights would soon go on in the surgery block and everything be prepared for an acute appendectomy.

Well remembered (except as to name) was the head porter, tall, ageing, gentle and ex-military. One of his duties was to sterilize the ambulance at the hospital door if it delivered an infectious case. This he did by means of a small formalin-filled spray-gun. I once arrived just as the ambulance was departing. I announced the new patient to be a case of scarlet fever. The porter grabbed his gun, raced after the ambulance and gave one squirt which fell short of the flapping back door by about six feet. He came back and said with satisfaction, 'By Jove, Sir, that was close. I nearly missed.'

I remember the girl of about eighteen whose appendix I had removed. She was all curls and simpers and her appendix was the most interesting feature about her. She came back to hospital a month later to thank me and assure me of her steady progress. A few weeks later she was back again, this time with her mother. On the next visit they treated it as a reunion of old friends. What did I do with my free week-ends, asked mother. Would I care to be their guest for a couple of days? Only a Taranaki dairy farm but I would be very welcome. Eileen would show me round. I would find the milking of cows very interesting. What about next week-end? Not next week-end, I said bluntly. My fiancée would be coming down from Hamilton then. I never saw them again.

As junior house surgeon I received one hundred pounds a year (and keep), and as senior one hundred and fifty pounds a year (same keep). In some hospitals junior house surgeons worked for fifty pounds a year and a few for nothing (except keep). My next target was general practice. In those days practices were usually acquired through the purchase of goodwill. Today they are acquired by the process of squatting. To buy a practice, with equipment and car would cost about two thousand pounds, and if I carefully saved half my present salary I would have the money in about twenty-five years. The period was too long. I finished at New Plymouth in 1927, bought a second-hand practice at Te Aroha and a second-hand car, went to Wellington, married (nothing second-hand there), borrowed from my father-in-law and up to Te Aroha we went, a team of two, confident of fame and fortune.

The miseries of the next two years can be briefly told. It was not till we got there that we met the Depression for the first time. In Te Aroha and round it, were shopkeepers, tradesmen, workmen, dairy farmers, go-as-you-please Maoris and Dalmation ditch-diggers from the Hauraki plains. They had two constant fears – unemployment and bankruptcy. In a district where there were two popular doctors and no need for more, there could only be one fate for a third. By this time I knew a lot about medicine but I knew nothing about medical practice. I was to learn that it was possible for a vendor of a practice to present highly satisfactory records of work done without revealing that they represented work done for another doctor when sick; or that the goodwill of a practice does not exist as a drifting cloud or a spiral of smoke; or that a declared overhaul of a car may not have got further than the speedometer.

For the first fortnight I sat in my expensive rooms in the theatre block without seeing a single patient. Then a woman, looking for Dr Dempster who had just departed, came to me. The next week she brought a friend and the following week another friend. Each paid ten shillings and sixpence. This, if represented on a graph, was heartening – the curve was shooting up, but if the graph was replaced with a balance sheet I was earning less than thirty pounds a year. Then quite suddenly I developed a monopoly of practice in Clarkin's quarry where lived many Maoris in houses of packing cases and galvanized iron. My frequent calls there were all optimistically recorded. Dr Lawrence warned me, 'They'll never accept your treatment. The really sick ones are taken down the line to the Pah. And they will never pay you.' In this last he was wrong. One Maori did pay me ten and six. It was in the street on a Saturday evening and he was very drunk. His attempt to recover it on the Monday morning failed because it had already been spent.

121

For what they were worth other artifices were tried. 'Drive like hell,' was the counsel of Dr Leatham, radiologist at New Plymouth. 'If you're only going to the library for a book, drive like hell.' So I drove like hell but no one was deceived. It was one of those places just cosy enough to know everyone else's business and there was no difficulty in knowing mine, what there was of it. Socially we had more success. We made many friends, some of whom persisted for years. I wrote (anonymously) a weekly column for the local paper. It comprised light prose and verse mainly about old identities, my information coming secretly from two old identities themselves. The circulation of the paper rose. Te Aroha was amused but puzzled. One of our friends, a voluble spinster, used to visit us weekly and explain the jokes. For this I received one pound a week which in terms of bread and butter in the Depression was not to be despised. I became secretary of the Savage Club and then their president–elect.

Sorry as this story is, it was not unique. The wisest of the young doctors in those days were those who stayed in hospital and never had to face the possibility of penury. In two more years, lawyers, engineers, teachers and dentists were to be found working on the roads. I doubt if any doctors did that but there must have been some narrow escapes. At the present time most of the profession prefers its income to be based on the private fees of patients. It is a view that ignores the lessons of history.

We lived precariously on borrowed money, on occasional writing, on a trickle of patients, on life insurance fees (travelling round the country with the agent), and on the generosity of Dr Lawrence. It is necessary to linger a little over Dr Lawrence. He was tall, ungainly, but a dedicated doctor. He worked tirelessly day and night over town and country. In a little cottage hospital across the river, he often did major surgery. He was a member of nearly all the clubs and societies in the place and frequently adjusted a bad balance sheet with a cheque.

He did all he could to help me: deflected some patients to me, sent me on some long country calls pretending they were emergencies, and used me as anaesthetist. Sometimes I would arrive for a minor anaesthetic and find the case finished, with Lawrence full of apologies for misquoting the time and the matron who was a good anaesthetist saying nothing. For all these he insisted on paying me. For thirty-six years Dr Lawrence was the servant of Te Aroha. In 1952 he received the M.B.E. Higher decorations have often been given with less cause.

Comparable in skill and merit was Dr George Home of New Plymouth. He was a brilliant surgeon, a splendid teacher and the most helpful of colleagues. During the war the famous trio of surgeons at Walton-on-Thames comprised Acland of Christchurch, Wyllie of

Palmerston North and Home of New Plymouth. The last was known as the 'BIPP king', from his development of the technique of fusing BIPP (bismuth – iodoform – paraffin paste) which was a very useful product in the days before antibiotics. He had one characteristic and well-remembered pose: sitting on the edge of a table after some midnight operation, waiting for his cup of tea and reciting volubly from Gilbert and Sullivan.

Occasional success at Te Aroha only accentuated the general failure. A few of Lawrence's patients began to come to me. He said he was delighted but no doctor, large-hearted though he may be, can be delighted at the defection of his friends. Nor could I be happy with such patients. It was plain after eighteen months that I had no future in Te Aroha.

As if to confirm this there appeared an advertisement in an Auckland paper inviting applications for a Medical Association practice at Blackball on the West Coast of the South Island. For several days we discussed it. Testimonials would be necessary. I approached a prominent business man with whom I was friendly. Would he do me a favour?

'Sorry, old man, I'm afraid I can't. The way things are . . . .'

'But you don't know what I want.'

'Well, you want to borrow money, don't you?'

'No, I do not want to borrow money.'

'Oh, sorry, my mistake. What is it then?'

'Doesn't matter.'

Even though I had never borrowed money in Te Aroha itself this was apparently my image. Time to get out, more than time to get out.

It was a most careful letter of application, written three times. There may have been a few judicious omissions but there was no statistical fact that would not survive in a court of law. I was very conscious that the letter had to go before a committee of miners. I tried to anticipate their philosophy and to some extent must have succeeded, for the application was approved over forty-eight others.

So here I was, getting out of the goods train at Otira and just in front, dry under a tarpaulin, was my brand new Essex. For this I had to thank my good friends the N.Z. Insurance Co. who had arranged the railing and paid the freight and had motored me to Otira and had offered me twenty-five pounds a year for signing the accident certificates of the Blackball miners. Gladly I accepted such largesse and after it was too late, became aware that it precluded me from claiming the one pound per case that the law provided for each of the three hundred accidents a year in the mine. Simple Simon indeed.

My wife and the six-month-old baby were with her parents in Wellington, waiting on my report. I had no money, no assets, and debts so formidable that I dared not add them up. But, unlike thousands in that deepening Depression, I had a job.

The tarpaulin was dragged off the car which was then run down a ramp into the mud. I climbed in. The mountains and the forest pressed all round and the rain cascaded down. Somewhere in the wilderness ahead, so the secretary of the Blackball Medical Association, one Hunter Ritchie, had informed me, was a roof and five hundred pounds a year. I studied the map and set out. The car slithered in the mud, the rain slashed the windscreen.

But, unknown at the time, that was the day I passed out of the tunnel – not the tunnel of Otira, which was merely a symbol, but the long tunnel of vicissitude.

'Go straight ahead,' the man with the tarpaulin had said, not knowing where I was going. The car, skidding and humping, went straight ahead. The rain switched off at Kumara where, so I had heard, every second house displayed a picture of Dick Seddon. The rain resumed again at Greymouth, a place I found impressive, partly for its size and partly because it was there at all. In the wild disorder of the coast every intrusion of civilization is surprising. Up the Grey Valley the rain stopped again and filmy mists were pegged out along the blue mountain sides.

I turned off at Ngahere. Blackball is pinched between the river and the ranges, is not on the road to anywhere and was then linked to the wider world by a creaking wooden bridge. I crossed it and climbed the hill beyond. The approach to the town was guarded by the cemetery. I turned into the main street.

It was less of a street than a rough road with deep ditches on either side. The houses were small, unpainted and all with tarred roofs. Weeds were often window-high and the scrub and gorse filled the many vacant sections. Yet, the houses stood out starkly because of the sparseness of trees. Halfway up on the left was a street of high rusted pylons, relics of an earlier aerial railway for coal.

At the top of the hill was a hotel, a shop or two round the corner. I asked for the doctor's house. 'Go straight on,' said the man at the hotel. It was five-roomed and was prominent because it was painted and had a detached surgery. An old man peered at me from the surgery door. This was the locum. I explained myself and he was suddenly animated. 'Then I can catch the four o'clock bus. See that house over there? The woman there is very sick. You had better see her tonight. The committee's coming to meet you at five. They'll tell you everything. Here's the key. Good luck.'

The waiting room was square with wooden seats nailed round three sides. A passage past a storeroom led to the surgery, where two walls had shelving to the ceiling all packed with bottles. Electric sterilizer,

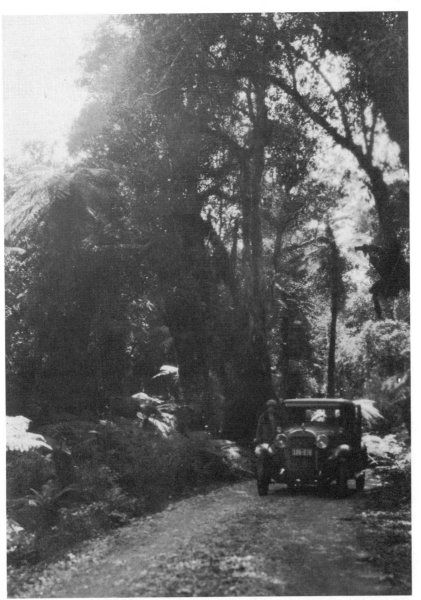

'My brand-new Essex', West Coast, 1928

dispensary scales, a horsehair couch, a hand basin, fireplace . . . . The essentials were there, but it was stark and austere. There was nothing to linger over. I went into the house. Small rooms, some recently painted, a kitchen of the simplest with a massive coal range. The water supply was from the roof. An outhouse sat over a deep pit. There was a shed at the back of the section, and a wash-house and coalhouse near the back door. There was no garden. The path from the gate to the surgery was of concrete. Most other paths anywhere were of crushed cinders.

The committee came at five; Hunter Ritchie, Snowy Cruse, Hutchinson, Bromilow, Mountford, possibly others. They were serious middle-aged men in good suits with white shirts and no collars.

They welcomed me to Blackball. I expressed appreciation at my appointment. They asked a few questions and I replied with others. They tried a joke or two and so did I. We were all more amused than was justified. We confirmed the existing surgery hours. They produced a contract which I was to study that night and to sign in the morning. We parted with a goodwill just hearty enough to be a little artificial. Each party was trying to sum up the other. Each at the moment could return only an open verdict.

I studied the agreement. I was to promise free medical attention to members of the Association which included the miners and their families at the Blackball mine and at the Paparoa mine, a few miles further on. There was a right to private practice with twenty-five pounds a year deducted for medicine supplied to private cases, midwifery two pounds ten shillings a case, miscarriages one pound ten, teeth extraction two and six a tooth with anaesthetic, one shilling without. Salary five hundred pounds a year.

I accepted the contract. Even though they were telling me what to do they could not tell me how to do it. I did not look hard for points to dispute for I had had no previous experience of five hundred pounds a year.

I went to the hotel, booked in, had an early meal and went back to pay my first visit on the sick woman. In addition to her advanced congestive heart failure due to mitral stenosis, she was pregnant, a hopeless combination. I strongly advised terminating the pregnancy. Just as firmly she and her husband refused. Two months later she died.

I went back to the surgery and at the right time turned on all the lights. About a dozen patients came. Their complaints in the main were either trivial or artificial, but their curiosity was high. I sensed that their impressions would soon be the property of everyone. I pretended a gaiety I did not feel and succeeded in making some of them laugh – a subtle defence against criticism. The last to come in was a pleasant middle-aged man who introduced himself as secretary of a Lodge. After a little he said, 'Well, here's the list and the money. Just sign the receipt here.' He gave me thirty-five pounds. I had no idea I was entitled to Lodge fees. I thought it was an annual sum but the next night when the other Lodge secretary arrived and paid me twenty-five pounds I learned that both sums were quarterly.

Nevertheless, that night I wrote to my wife in total disparagement of the whole project. I stressed the soot, the sulphurous smell, the lack of trees, of paint, of a telephone, a library, a hospital, a garage. It was just a place where people existed. The people themselves seemed friendly enough but that was not enough. I intended staying just long enough to earn the money to get out. Together we would find somewhere else. In the meanwhile she had better stay in Wellington. Don't waste money on fares.

Having posted this letter I went across the road to the hotel. The door was locked but I heard the hubbub of many people. I knocked loudly. Immediately the noise ceased. After a little the door opened a few degrees. Inside was Tom Gilmore, manager for the proprietress, Mrs Campbell. He recognised me and flung the door wide. 'Oh, it's you, Doctor. Look, never knock on the front door again. Go round the back like a gentleman.' He yelled out, 'All right, boys. It's only the Doc.' The lights came on, the doors opened, the noise resumed. I was passed along a chain of introduction, crushing handshakes, noisy welcomes, beer and jocularity. I had a drink. 'Never drink with your patients,' Sir Lindo Ferguson had advised. He should have added, 'Never make your professional debut in a Blackball pub after hours.'

Campbell's hotel was a square wooden double-storeyed building and without any subtleties of architecture or facilities. After six p.m. all patrons, like gentlemen, went to the back door with the exception of the local constable, who was also like a gentleman in that he knocked on the door exactly at six-fifteen, and if he was a little early didn't mind waiting. The back door led into an atmosphere, warm, both literally and domestically. The gentlemen often served themselves at meals, helped the barman at rush periods, sat on the corner of the kitchen table and argued with the cook and generally turned the hotel into a home at no extra cost.

My wife, having been ordered to stay away, arrived at Stillwater by the first available train. She favoured Blackball more than I did. The baby seemed delighted with it. Pending our near departure we ordered some skimpy furniture.

We stayed nearly five years. They were the happiest years of our lives.

The heart of Blackball was the mine and its lifeblood was coal. Neither town nor mine could exist apart. All day and all night there were miners on the move: front shift, back shift and dogwatch. All through the town could be heard the racket of the bins, the rattle of the trucks, the salvage of one thousand tons of coal a day and every morning at dawn the rumble of the long long Christchurch coal train. Blackball was a 'safe' mine, which meant that there was no firedamp (carburetted hydrogen) and the men used acetylene lamps. There was much black damp (carbon dioxide), a gas so heavy that a candle burning brightly at one level might be extinguished two inches lower. Yet Paparoa, a few miles up in the hills, was not a safe mine. I was called one day to an explosion when there had been only two men in the mine. They were lying ten or twelve feet from the mine entrance stripped of all clothing with their whole bodies charred black.

The miner on the coal face may be half a mile underground in a small box-like space, hot, artificially ventilated and connected to the living world by a series of narrow tunnels all vulnerable to geophysical forces. The coal face disintegrates before his pick or his blasting. Then it is shovelled into trucks. This shovelling is the main part of a miner's life and is heavy, unimaginative, exclusively physical. Two men work to a truck, shovelling about, left right, left right, massive and muscular, pausing for a moment when the trucker changes trucks but rarely pausing otherwise for they are paid by output. It is a struggle they never win. Always ahead of them is the coal face. Each may lift on his shovel thirty tons of coal a day. Twenty or thirty years later he may still be trying to lift thirty tons a day. There are no colours on the coal face, no target for ambition, no easing of effort, unless he becomes a deputy or even a mine manager. These rarely tempt for they involve examinations and a subtle change in ideology. He remains therefore in step with the pit pony, the oxen treading out the corn, the bullock under the yoke. It is dangerous work. The hazards are falls of coal, earthquakes, the eruption of an underground river, the failure of the fan, poisonous gases and explosions. He survives through knowledge and vigilance. In my first week I was taken down the mine on a guided tour. In one claustrophobic hole I was invited to test the security of the roof. I swung the pick as instructed. There was an ominous booming sound. I dropped the pick and raced for the entrance, amid much amusement. Yet, a little later in another place they all suddenly rushed for the main drive, two of them sweeping me along. Behind us there fell about a ton of coal from the roof.

The hazards of mining are illustrated by a quiet retired deputy who consulted me once about some deep grazes on his arm. All that he would tell me was that he had fallen on some coal. His mates later told me more. The previous night he and two others had been driving a tramway downhill taking out the coal and timbering up as they went. Suddenly there was a shout from above. The rake of trucks they had just sent up had broken loose and was now rushing down in the dark. The tunnel they were in was no more than six feet high. It was wide enough for the truck only. The deputy's reaction was the reflex of an experienced miner. Two recesses, about a foot deep, had been cut into the walls for the supporting wooden pillars. He pressed each of his mates into one of these. For himself he grasped a cross beam and judging the appropriate moment by the sound swung his body up to the roof as an athlete circles the bar. Below him the trucks smashed against the wall and he dropped down on the wreckage, grazing his arm. The three of them spent the rest of the shift clearing up the mess.

My second descent into the mine was at the end of my first fortnight and followed a summons, not an invitation. The secretary of the Miners' Union had been drilling for a shot and had not heard the warning from the roof. He was crushed and buried. At the end of the drive I met his mates trudging uphill with the stretcher. I gave an injection of morphine using some cold tea as a solvent (on other occasions I used water leaking through the roof). When he was examined at home he had at least seven fractures. The shock was massive and he died in a few hours.

Death is always trailing the miner quite apart from the major disasters. (Kaitangata 1879, thirty-five dead; Brunner 1896, sixty-seven dead and in 1926 another nine; Huntly 1914, forty-three dead and in 1939, eleven dead.) Invalidity and premature death following accidents, early heart failure, silicosis, pneumonia, chronic bronchitis, emphysema and premature ageing are all hazards of mining but do not get in the mining statistics. Later preventive legislation has reduced the incidences, but no legislation can wholly protect against the acts of God and the mistakes of man.

But there is no compulsion. Any miner can leave the mine and a few do. Of the rest the phrase 'Once a miner, always a miner' applies. He comes back to the mine again and again. His children succeed him on the coal face. I have questioned miners about this addiction, but their explanations leave the question unanswered. 'It is all I can do.' 'I am settled here.' Perhaps there is a satisfaction in invading the heart of a mountain and tearing down pillars of coal where there has been silence and immobility for millions of years; perhaps, because he is usually a rebel against many aspects of the social system he prefers to argue from a common background; perhaps through mining he maintains the bond with his friends and the community's social standard.

Politics were simple in Blackball. The class warfare kept surging, the battle plans having been drawn up by Karl Marx. The battle flags were black or white, with rarely a hint of grey. They were so fervently uncompromising that many protests became inevitable. Karl Marx, I argued, was wrong. In the world of industry compromise and not confrontation was now the key. Both parties in mutual trust and confidence should concede . . . .

'It's a hundred years too late for that sort of stuff, Doc. D'you know what they have done to us?'

Actually I did not. Most of them or their ancestors had been miners in Scotland, Northern England and a few from Wales. Their tales would have been verbally perpetuated down the generations and may well have outgrown the truth. I wanted a more reliable source and found in Trevelyan's *Illustrated English Social History, Vol. III* (London, Longmans, 1951) a report on Scottish mines:

> This iniquitous system of serfage was abolished at the end of the Eighteenth Century. Till then, the Scottish miner, together with his wife and children who carried up the coal he cut, were transferable with the pit on any change of proprietorship. They could not leave their employment during life.

And in *Volume IV*:

> The revelation of the appalling conditions of female and child labour in the coal-mines, an evil several centuries old, had led to Lord Shaftesbury's Mines Act of 1842, by which the underground employment of women and children under ten was forbidden. By an Act of 1850 adult males were also protected by a Mines Inspectorate . . . .

The miners' capitalist employers saw little and cared less about their conditions of life and labour.

But that was old history, though it was still remembered among the miners. More recent history was that the Blackball mine had opened in 1893. Fifteen years later the Blackball miners were on strike. They demanded half an hour for lunch instead of the allotted fifteen minutes. The Company refused and the strike lasted eleven weeks. There was much hardship but, as so often in strikes, a principle was at stake. The miners won but the Union was fined seventy-five pounds for striking. In the course of the hearing the judge voiced his opinion that fifteen minutes was enough for lunch. Shortly after, it being then midday, he adjourned the court till two p.m. The Union refused to pay the fine and their personal chattels were seized – bedroom furniture, kitchen equipment, sewing machines, bicycles – and were publicly auctioned in the street. The total sum realized was twelve and sixpence and the goods were returned to the original owners.

It could hardly be described as a vicious strike but it was important. The

Blackball miners had amused the country at the expense of the Company and were now ready to press on. A New Zealand Federation of Miners followed, changing its title the next year to the Federation of Labour. Thereafter Blackball led other unions in dogged political campaigning. From this and the neighbouring mines there came a nationwide influence. Webb and Hickey both worked in the Blackball mine and Semple worked nearby.

The relations between the Company and the Union were appalling. On the Union's side it was a deep implacable hatred. The Company's attitude was unknown. Its representatives came to Blackball only at intervals of a few years when the contract would need renewing. They would pick their way through the cinders to the miners' hall and there confronting the executive across the table would thrash out a new agreement and then make for their car at the door.

I resumed my argument. 'But why the bitterness? What has the Company done?'

'What has it done? It has beaten us down to the last penny. What else has it done? Nothing.'

This last was dismally true. The Company paid the wages and nothing more. It was a town were there were a thousand opportunities for making some gesture of goodwill. When I first motored up the main street I had been struck by what seemed to be civic neglect. It was a wrong judgement. All the town possessed in the way of amenities – medical association, doctor, domain, football team, football grounds, swimming baths, miners' hall and pictures twice a week, debating clubs, sickness fund – had come from a scraping off the wages. No amenity could be traced to the Company. The miners quoted to me the old man who was putting in a shot when a deputy pulled the wrong lever and blew the charge out in his face. He was permanently blinded. There was no compensation and the Company paid him up to the half-shift when he was injured. Thereafter he lived on the sixpences taken for many years out of each miner's pay packet.

It was hard for the miner to imagine a neutral attitude. The mine manager, the mine engineer and secretary, the school teacher, postmaster and doctor were automatically on the side of the capitalist. We could still all be good friends but politically could not be trusted. I gave grim evidence of this on my second day.

Of the hundred or more single miners who were under notice of dismissal at the end of the month, forty-two had cajoled my indulgent predecessor into signing them up for compensation. They arrived in a bunch on the traditional morning for compensation cases. The green form each brought asked two questions: was the bearer fit for work and when would he be? I did not realize that these were alternatives. I answered both stating that the bearer was not fit for work but would be in one week, ten days, two weeks. . . . I intended to see them all again and perhaps modify the dates. But a date quoted was a date finalized. In the mine office they began making up the final pay packets. The town, I understood later, was seething. On the first morning the new doctor had signed off thirty-eight men as fit for work, well knowing that there was no work. He was obviously in the pay of the Company (wrong, I have never in my life had any dealings with the Company). He was on the payroll of the Insurance Company (correct, twenty-five pounds a year). He was politically an ultra-conservative (wrong, I had no politics then, though the seeds were being sown).

Fortunately, there arrived in the surgery on that same evening a middle-aged man who had hurt his knee in the mine and, because recovery was incomplete, he was offered a lump sum of twenty-five pounds in final settlement. He agreed to this but he had first to sign a form of release before a lawyer and a doctor. I refused. His knee was going to cripple him with gross osteo-arthritis. I was not going to fall a second time for a scandalous bribe of twenty-five pounds. I sent him to a Christchurch specialist, Mr J. Leslie Will, and he came back with a cheque for five hundred pounds. This bewildered Blackball. I was either a fool, blowing hot and cold, or a deep one, laying false trails. I was closely watched. Eventually I was granted the rare status of being an impartial adjudicator unbiased by politics. Proof of this was my regular appointment as judge of the baby show at the Labour Day sports.

The intransigence of the Blackball Company was well illustrated by the water supply. The miners relied on roof water, dirty with tar and soot. The galvanized tanks at the back of each house were empty in ten days. Thereafter the water was trucked from the Grey River at a shilling a bucket. But just above the pit head a tributary of the Blackball creek came tumbling down with clear mountain water, supplying the houses of the Company officials and the boilers and showers at the pit-head. To reticulate the town was an urgent public health need. I went to the committee of the Medical Association and they laughed, not at my idea, but at my enthusiasm. It was the same plan that they, through their Parliamentary representative, had been pushing for twenty years. 'Waste of time, Doctor, you'll get nothing out of them.' So I wrote to the Company pointing out that the water was there, the fall was right, the ditches for the pipes had already been dug. All that was needed was a mile and a half of pipes and the services of an engineer for a week. The miners would do the rest. The letter was not acknowledged. I was about to write to the Minister of Mines when the Minister himself (the Hon. A. J. Murdoch) arrived in person on some government business. Somehow I was involved. The minister said to me,

'You must find it depressing living in this place.'

'On the other hand I find it stimulating. At the moment I am trying to get a water supply installed. I was going to write to you inviting your co-operation.'

'Water supply? What water supply? I've heard nothing about a water supply.'

It was easy to tell him. From where he stood in front of the miners' hall I could point out the main landmarks, could produce a blueprint in air.

'Now this is very interesting,' he said. 'I have to go to a meeting just now but could we talk some more about this afterwards?'

Yes, we could. But we didn't. When I arrived punctually at our rendezvous he had already left town. I never saw him again.

When the secretary of the Miners' Union was killed, the Union took over the formalities and revealed that its role was with the living and had no rapport with the dead. It was a cold and menacing day as the funeral cortège went down the main street, the coffin carried by relays of miners. At the cemetery there was a pause till the stragglers arrived, then the coffin was lowered. Immediately two men with shovels began filling the grave with rocks, scoria and wet clay. There was no service, no speeches, no eulogy. At the end they all sang 'The Red Flag' but the wind caught the words and tossed them away. They went back up the street bent against the driving rain. There had been no work in the mine that day: the traditional homage to a man killed. Tomorrow the fans and the trucks and the screens would be noisy again and an emergency meeting would be called to elect a new secretary.

The miner found it hard to imagine a life that was not disciplined by a union.

'I wish our Union was as strong as yours, Doc.'

'You mean the B.M.A.? It's an association, not a union. We meet mainly to discuss better treatment opportunity.'

'Don't give us that stuff. . . . You all gotta belong, haven't you?'

'No, we please ourselves. Join or not as you like. Resign as you like.'

'That's not a union.'

'I know it isn't. It's an association.'

'Call it what you like. But it's really a union. Stands to reason. You're not a crowd of bloody fools. You've got a union all right.'

'It's an association. I ought to know. I belong to it.'

'So do the rest of you. You have another look at it, Doc. You'll find it's a union all right.'

The miner as a citizen was more attractive than the miner as a unionist. He was a staunch family man; a zealous custodian of his little cottage and its contents, a firm supporter of 'the missus' and proud of his children. Often he would be seen in the street with a child on his shoulder. His solicitude for a sick child was always sincere. 'Spare no expense,' he would insist, even though he would be living on credit before pay day. I once sent a boy of five or six to Greymouth hospital because of some puzzling neurological symptoms. Here a very young house-surgeon told the father a few days later that the child had meningitis and that he would die. The father, a flint-like character, well known for his intolerance of sentiment, religion and any social graces, was now a weak vessel of apprehension as he confronted me. He insisted I go to Greymouth and investigate. This I did the following day. The alleged meningitis was in fact meningism, which is unimportant. That night the father marched into the surgery and closed the door. I was sitting at my desk.

'You saw the boy?'

'Yes, I saw the boy. He's all right. He'll be home in a few days.'

For a few seconds he stared at me. Then he walked to the centre of the surgery, went down on his knees, removed his cap, bent forward in an attitude of devotion and said,

'Say that again, Doctor.'

'The boy's all right. He'll be home in a few days.'

Again there was the pause. Then he got to his feet, slapped his cap on his head and marched off without further words.

Despite the grey environment the miner put plenty of colour in his life. He had his beer or two after every shift, day or night. He played horseshoes with extraordinary skill and strength. And he was addicted to practical jokes. One of his number, famed for being horticulturally light-fingered, overheard a conversation and as a result became possessed of a bundle of rose cuttings from the station platform. The subsequent rose garden was viewed by everyone with interest and amusement till it became apparent that rose cuttings and blackberry cuttings are practically indistinguishable.

Another elderly man short in the breath as befitted his age and occupation blamed the Company for denying him access to good clean air. His mates bore with his obsession till he was cured by his personal invention. He fixed about a yard of half-inch conduit on the wall of the main drive down which the wind whistled and then twisted the last six inches at right angles so as to deliver fresh air under his nose as he sat in his cul-de-sac working his winch. He had no further trouble. Breathing was perfect. He was heartily congratulated by his mates, the same ones who had stuffed the pipe full of soft soap.

A miner once said to me:

'The baby, Doctor – he's pretty sick, isn't he? Well, the missus and I have been talking it over. We know you're doing your best but if you can't save him we'd like you to baptize him.' (The baby recovered: I insisted on it.)

I was once involved in a graceful ecumenical incident. On a certain Sunday morning a select group in the pub heard with indignation that the service in the little Presbyterian church was going to be cancelled because there was no organist. The normal organist was a miner who played with all stops out. At the moment he was under restraint at the police station, having incurred the constable's displeasure the night before by emphasizing his political views by means of a walking stick on the head of his opponent. The bar patrons disagreed with the constable. It was a bloody shame to stop whatever they wanted to do down at the church because of a walking stick. It was a clear case for an umpire. So they drained their glasses and came up to see me. Would I intervene with the policeman? So I intervened. The policeman was reasonable and was also a grateful patient. The prisoner was brought in and some mighty oaths were sworn. He then went up the road and played lustily. Back at the police station the constable's wife had a hot dinner waiting for him. The singing was heard up at the pub where the protest group nodded in approval. They were as indifferent to religion as a new-born babe. I, for census purposes, was a Presbyterian and the constable was a Roman Catholic. The organist was of dubious faith but some of his ancestors had been Methodists. The congregation was composed of anyone who was prepared to come. An appropriate hymn would have been 'Onward Christian Soldiers'.

Though I eventually became accepted at Blackball this was not based on clinical ability. I rose or fell in favour not by diagnosis but by deeds. I was helped considerably by three separate incidents.

Down the main road, in the house of her married daughter, lived an old lady regarded as a high suicide risk. She had once attempted drowning in the Grey River and for years her family had watched her day and night with all knives and sharp instruments locked away. I saw her, a silly old hysteric revenging herself on her daughter for having got married. On my advice they left the knife drawer open, put a couple of bottles of coloured water marked 'Poison' on the dresser, added a coil of rope on the back porch and gave her free access to the Grey River. And, on the first occasion when there were adequate spectators, she stumbled off to the river, waded in up to her knees, faced the shore and yelled, 'Help, help'. No one stirred. At last she was forced to wend her sulky way home. Through this incident I acquired many friends and one enemy.

The second episode began at four a.m. with a man knocking on my front door. He was Mr P. Coates, a famous name on the Coast. He was dripping wet, having swum the Ahaura River in the dark. He had come from the Kopara, an isolated farming area thirty miles away in the foothills of the Alps. There were only two families there, Parkinson and Mallinson. Parkinson was sick – abdominal pains and vomiting – and Mr Mallinson thought he had an acute appendix. This was a comfort because the lay diagnosis of abdominal conditions is always wrong. It was, said my informant, utterly impossible to get him out. The rivers were in high flood after a week's rain, there were no bridges and the bush track into the place was quagmire.

The first half of the journey was in the comfort of the car; where the bush track commenced, two youths on ponies were waiting, with a spare horse for me. Each took one of my two bags. The horse, slipping down banks and clambering up the other side, seemed unaware that it had a passenger. When, in the late morning, I dismounted at the gate to the farmhouse yard, the horse looked round at me in surprise. Inside the house were all the local inhabitants, worried yet grateful. Their worry was soon transferred to me, for the patient undoubtedly had an acute appendix and in the days before antibiotics was certainly going to die unless a surgeon intervened. I verified from them all that transport was impossible. They had proved the day before that the patient could not now mount a horse.

There was no alternative to surgery. Before the patient was carried to the kitchen table where the operation was planned, I made him make his will which I signed. He had a private word one by one with his family. But in the end it was the comedy which predominated.

I selected Mrs Mallinson as anaesthetist. I put it to her and she paled, swayed and I caught her as she fell. So I turned to her husband, a tough old farmer of over sixty, grounded in common sense. It was, he said, not much in his line but he would do what he could. The sterilizer was a kerosene tin swinging over an open fire. It was taken outside and after it had been drained through holes punched in the bottom it was set in a wide milk pan by the operating table. Having no gown I boiled up one of Mrs Parkinson's aprons and it dissolved and left a slimy sludge on all my instruments. These were not many. One of my four artery forceps dropped on the floor in the early stages. For swabs there was boiled up a pound of cotton wool, paper and all. Having no carbolic I sterilized the appendix stump with pure sheep dip.

The surgical details do not matter. The operation was slow mainly because it was almost extravagantly cautious. But at last the abdomen was firmly sewn up and on the patient's chest was a turgid appendix in a saucer. Mr Mallinson, taking over the ether bottle after I had induced the patient, gave a magnificent anaesthetic, better than many I have done. The patient was cleared out to his bedroom and we sat down to an excellent roast dinner which had been cooked in the stove in the far wall of the theatre, by the patient's wife tip-toeing in and out with averted gaze. I left morphia and a syringe and written instructions. I wrote a note of explanation to the owner of the farm (Mr Heaphy of Greymouth) and entrusted it to one of my bush escorts who was going into Greymouth. Then after another hazardous crossing of the swirling Kopara River I finally reached the car and home.

There were consequences. Mr Heaphy, in collaboration with Dr Moore, sent out a nurse and equipment, and when I went back a few days later the professional array was intimidating. Mr Mallinson was immediately christened 'Doc Mallinson'. The operation was exploited by local bodies to get a government grant for roads and bridges, and new settlers began to arrive. In cases of sickness they usually went to Doc Mallinson, arguing that no man could have a title like that without good reason. Some weeks later a man from that district said in my surgery:

'You must be the doctor who operated on poor old Parkinson.'

I sat up. 'What's wrong with him?'

'Haven't you heard? He's in bed, can't move hardly.'

Immediately all the black catastrophies came leaping at me. Slipped ligature, chronic pelvic sepsis, subphrenic abscess. . .?

'But what has happened?'

'Pitched off his horse he was. They thought at first his leg was broken. Doc Mallinson put him to bed.'

My absence from Blackball on that Good Friday had not been noticed, there being no surgery hours. On the Monday the *Grey River Argus* told the whole story in detail, ignoring the surgical aspects and dwelling on the cowboy attributes. It was grossly inaccurate but very amusing. The story came to Blackball by means of the paper, and, I have no doubt, had considerable conversational value for twenty-four hours. It would of course be critically examined, but it had no political overtones, had harmed nobody and had proved that the doctor was capable when necessary of some initiative. The verdict therefore was of approval.

The third episode is recounted with reluctance. It concerned a young miner who was noted for his aggressive views and general bravado. This tended to cover his insecurity for being unable to read or write. He relied heavily on the Union and also on the Communist Party. There were few communists in Blackball but he was one, and in any political argument would reverse the lapel of his coat to show the badge.

He came into the surgery one evening. He had hurt his back in the mine. The history was not convincing, the symptoms were bizarre and the examination negative. I disssmissed him with some words of reassurance. The next morning he returned. The back was worse. He couldn't bend. (I later accidentally/intentionally swept a paper knife off the table at his feet and he stooped and picked it up.) He demanded to be signed on compensation. His story had shifted; so had his symptoms. If his back had deteriorated so had my credulity. I recommended that he go to work in the morning.

Instead he returned the next day noisy and truculent. He demanded his papers. Otherwise he would report me to the Medical Association which would immediately dismiss me. He refused to let me examine his back again. Bloody nonsense. A proper doctor would have known the first time. I told him that, unfortunately for him, a proper doctor had; that I did not believe his story which was obviously manufactured, that he was getting no compensation, that my waiting room was full and the sooner he left the sooner I could deal with them.

He put his back against the door. He refused to get out. The surgery belonged to the Medical Association, not to me. He had a better right to be there than I had. He had half a mind to order me out.

I stood up. 'Get out.'

'I'm not getting out.'

'Get out or I'll put you out.'

He was probably not as astonished at this threat as I was. The words had been born out of the situation and had no considered volition. I had no wish to smear the professional image by brawling with patients. But this was Blackball where the professional image was not recognized but a man was expected to be a man for a' that. If I let myself be intimidated by him I would never be more than a second-rate doctor.

'You put me out,' he sneered. I moved up to him and he stepped back. I followed. He put out his fists defensively. With both hands I grasped his right wrist, swung him round and forced his arm up behind his back. I was angry and put on the pressure. He cried out with pain but I had him powerless. It was no skill on my part but merely luck with the advantage of surprise. With my free hand I opened the surgery door and then transferred it to the seat of his pants and marched him out and down the short corridor in front of the storeroom. I stepped up the momentum and when his heels slipped on the polished linoleum I gave him a final shove and he slid across the waiting room to the door. I went back and locked the surgery door. It had been a disturbing incident. I was apprehensive about the consequences. Eventually when I had settled somewhat I opened the surgery door. But the waiting room was empty.

I waited and, sure enough, the secretary of the Medical Association arrived later. But he was extraordinarily affable. He wanted to know how I was getting on, or whether there was anything the Association could do for me. And though for several days I waited for the blow to fall, I seemed to be greeted everywhere with an amused amiability.

Eventually I was told the true story. One miner mentioned to another that he was going up to the surgery to get signed off for a back injury. Easy enough, said the second one. That doctor would fall for any story. The first one disagreed. If he wasn't convinced, that doctor could be tough. An argument developed and was resolved, as so many arguments were, in the pub. The bet was for five pounds and to win it, the second man had to be put on compensation for an alleged injured back. Within two hours the money was held by a referee and the witnesses were sworn to secrecy. The man with the intact back came to the surgery and within the forty-eight hour period was thrown out.

It was a story which in Blackball was regarded as particularly rich even though it was the old set scene of the deflation of an agent. It had a short life, of course, in its original form. When miners of two different mines met in a neutral pub the story became beer-garnished and barely recognizable. My main characteristics, said the patrons from Blackball, were sympathy with the genuine, and the ejection of the imposter. Every time the story was told the malingerer travelled further through space before landing.

In my second year the West Coast Unions had the right to appoint their own medical officer to the Miners' Phthisis Pensions Appeal Board in Christchurch and they appointed me.

In that there was no town council, no mayor, no civic authority, the Union when necessary assumed their functions. During the 1918 influenza epidemic the Union placed an armed guard on the bridge, which was the only way in and out. Anyone could leave Blackball but no one could enter it. Blackball had no influenza during the epidemic. Though the Union had its own method of disciplining those who trespassed against its rules or its political philosophy (to be branded a scab was a dreadful sentence of life-long ignominy), yet it resisted any legislative intrusion on personal freedom. When, after the war, compulsory military training was re-introduced into schools, a uniformed First Lieutenant arrived at the Blackball school and put some of the senior boys through their first drill.

As he left he met a deputation of miners. They led him to the cliff above the Grey River and indicated that the rocks below would be his final destination if he appeared in the place again. Thereafter Blackball was the invariable victim of the shortage of military staff in Greymouth.

Some miners volunteered during the war and went overseas with full Union approval. (Mining was a protected industry.) But the Union did not approve of the compulsion of conscription and was well known for favouring deserters. When the police arrived seeking such men the latter would soon be on the long winding tracks up the Paparoa range, where they could look down on Blackball and be informed of all the movements of the police through the code of specially arranged sheets and towels on certain trees. There was some deference shown to old Mrs Frickleton who lived in the little cottage behind the hotel, because her son had the V.C., but there was more pride in Nick Peterson, a harmless miner of German origin, because he had escaped from Somes Island by swimming and had come back to Blackball to resume coal production for British ships. Peterson was kindly and innocuous and was formidable only on the chess board as I verified on a number of sad occasions.

The unionists were fundamentally honest. Law and order in Blackball was represented by one co-operative constable and an unwritten community spirit. I knew of no major thefts, no scandals, no violence (beyond a bare-fisted encounter now and then in a circle of twenty or so referees with two of them holding the stakes), no vandalism and no vagrancy. Can any city suburb with twelve hundred inhabitants say the same?

Just as Blackball was an odd place so were its diseases. For instance in five years there were no cases of cancer. They were not overlooked for they are woefully obvious in the final stages. According to national statistics there should have been twenty-three. Why should this be? The air was full of the by-products of coal which are a rich source of carcinogens. Why the immunity?

The same air was probably responsible for the high incidence of asthma. There were thirty-five asthmatics in a radius of half a mile from the surgery, most of them miners. Their only remedy was adrenalin and some stramonium cigarettes. They showed a peculiar pattern in that a large group would all suffer an acute attack together with no obvious personal, meteorological or other discernible reason. Some unknown factor was at work, probably in the mine. The circumstances provided a splendid opportunity for research. I planned an investigation but required some equipment costing a few pounds only. My application for government help drifted between the Mines Department and the Health Department for nearly two years. Periodically someone would write from Wellington to ask why I wanted the apparatus. Eventually the matter was disposed of by Dr Fletcher Telford, Medical Officer of Health for Canterbury and Westland. Through the local Member (Mr H. Holland) I saw his report which was to the effect that he had been Medical Officer at Blackball years before, that he knew the conditions well and that no research on asthma was justifiable.

This rejection of an earnest investigation would never have happened now. Certainly the times were unpropitious. The Depression was deepening, the Forbes Government brooded ineffectively over the country and Dr Telford did not have a research mind. (I once heard him at a B.M.A. meeting advocating unpasteurized milk.)

Sepsis was constant: boils, carbuncles, quinsies, pulp infections, suppurative tenosynovitis. Yet, though puerperal sepsis was rife at the time all through New Zealand, there were only two puerperal patients with a mild temperature among my five hundred confinements in Blackball and Ngahere. The conditions were excellent for gross sepsis. All the confinements were domiciliary and usually a few hours after the baby was born the front room was open to family traffic again. The nurses were always untrained neighbours who had never heard of asepsis.

An alternative to asthma research was an investigation of the anaemias of pregnancy. I had a microscope and the apparatus for blood counts. I began to investigate the blood as a routine in all cases, particularly after I left Blackball. The results eventually formed the basis of an M.D. thesis.

General practice in Blackball always had special features.

She came from Bell Hill, with her cat in her arms. They were both elderly and devoid of attraction, she because of her impregnable self-confidence, and her cat because it was dying of gangrene and it stank. Could I do anything for her darling cat? Could I give it an injection? I could and did, conveniently disposing of considerable unwanted drugs. And could I give her something for her nerves? I made up a bromide mixture. A few days later I received a note: 'My darling cat died in my arms at Ngahere.' I was not surprised. Had its nine lives been intact they would all have fallen before the contents of that syringe. 'I have not taken the tonic. There were a lot of crystals at the bottom of the bottle and as they looked like arsenic I thought I had better not take the risk.'

My obstetric practice was exacting. I had to carry in my bag the resources of a hospital and if the bag was missing or had not been replenished the only thing left was ingenuity. I have conducted a confinement in the back seat of a car and in a house where the only furniture was a wire mattress rushed in from a neighbour. I have tied an umbilical cord with my shoelace and have administered an enema with half a stethoscope. I also had a limited veterinary practice. I was called once to a labouring cow on a vacant section, ringed about by fifty interested spectators. From the knowledge of bovine obstetrics gained at Fairview I gave my opinion that the labour was hard but normal; let nature take its course and the calf would probably be born early tomorrow. This must have been overheard by the cow for it calved ten minutes later.

He came into the surgery easily compelling attention by his bland announcement that he was going to shoot his neighbour because his neighbour had poisoned his dog. It was a most valuable dog (most dead dogs are). Frisking on the chain when its owner went to work, dead on his return. The inference was obvious, but would I verify it by doing a post-mortem? I demurred and quoted many of the causes of canine death. But after two days he was unmoved by my medical terms and more determined on murder. So I had to meet his terms and do the post-mortem. This in itself was an experience, disputing with the flies the right of access to a dog lying dead for three days in the sun. The stomach was empty, the mucosa normal. There had been no poison. From the forensic point of view the case was finished. But there was some fluid in the pelvis. Investigation led to the ileum where at a point about six inches from the end there was a perforation and through it there projected into the peritoneal cavity the intact head of a tapeworm and several proglottides. It was a pretty demonstration of human hydatids in the making. I should have sent the whole specimen to Professor Murray Drennan of the Medical School. My only excuse was that the dog had reached an intolerable degree of deadness. I reported my findings to the dog owner and lent him some books with diagrams of tapeworms. He returned them with the comment that he still thought the dog had died of poisoning. But there was no murder.

Paparoa mine with its little cluster of houses round the mine entrance at the end of the road was easy of access. But there was also a settlement of single men half-way up the mountain side. This was known as Soldiers. Here had lived, ten years before, a trucker who was later to be Sir Francis Chichester. A call to Soldiers was to be dreaded for the track was steep and half an hour long. On one occasion a drunken miner hearing his mate cough, started a chain of communication, as a result of which I, carrying my black bag, arrived at two a.m., soaked to the skin in a vain search for a patient. Whenever possible patients from Soldiers were expected to come to me.

One such case prefaced his arrival late one night by inaugurating telephone calls at various points on his route urging me to stand by. I knew only that he was an accident case. Eventually he arrived not on a stretcher as I had expected but alone, marching in with noisy tread. In addition to being tall, dour, emotionless, he was also speechless. He would tell no tale, answer no questions and played the perfect role of the deaf mute. Just as bizarre were his trappings. A sapling down his back was fastened to his chest and abdomen with twine. To this was attached a right-angled arm splint and beneath this were smaller splints and smaller splints. Methodically, in a search for the lesion, I removed them one by one as if peeling an onion. Finally there was a matchbox splint holding an extended middle finger. On the finger across one knuckle was a scratch half an inch long and pin deep only. I covered the wound with a piece of sticking plaster the size of a large stamp, whereupon he turned on his heels, still speechless and marched off into the night. I never saw him again. But a few weeks later when some mountaineers were lost near Arthur's Pass he was, as a member of the rescue party, both valiant and reckless. A few weeks later he sent a box of poisoned chocolates through the post to a girl in Blackball. The wrong girl opened them, ate one and died. During the trial for murder he often turned his back on the court and indulged in hearty laughter. The jury's verdict was that he was insane. They would have known sooner if they had asked me.

There was a boy at Nelson Creek who took lunch to his father in the sawmill. His clothing got caught in a travelling belt. He was whirled away, flung against the ceiling, and dropped back among the machinery. . . . When I got there nearly an hour later the place was deserted. I was not surprised. I have seen men dismembered by bombs but this was worse. I got a clean sheet from his home. Half an hour later I sewed it up and gave orders that no one was to undo it.

'If you're passing today,' said a miner on the phone, 'would you drop in to see the baby? Nothing wrong, but the missus is worrying.' I arrived half an hour later. The family was in one corner of the room having breakfast. The cot was in the other corner. Both parents apologized for calling me. 'He's got a cold,' a piping five-year-old informed me. The baby was dead. Cot deaths give little warning.

Drama at Ahaura on a warm sunny afternoon with the schoolroom packed for an inquest. The victim had been a famished nine-month-old baby. Doctor, priest, and police had answered the original summons, but the constable had got there first and hence the inquest with a local jury of four and a J.P. as foreman. The mother gave tearful evidence of her vain search for a suitable food and her vain attempts to stop the vomiting. I (who had never seen the baby alive) gave evidence of malnutrition and starvation and at one stage unfortunately used the word 'marasmus'. This produced a sensation in court. I had to spell it, define it, enlarge on it. I offered to draw it, which confirmed the suspicion that something sinister was afoot. It became a tribunal, not so much concerned with the demise of a baby, as the integrity of a doctor. I was rigorously cross-examined by the constable who, among his ain folk, was having his crowded glorious hour. The jury deliberated for half an hour and then returned with the verdict that 'the baby died from what the doctor said'. These cases of verbal infanticide are extremely rare.

The most poignant of all tragedies in medicine are the tragedies of little children. There was the four-year-old at Ngahere who fell from a car; for four days no one knew that the broken rib had punctured the lung and on the fifth day she died; and the other little girl, aged three, also at Ngahere, whose nightdress caught fire one morning when her parents were out milking and whose four-year-old brother climbed on a table and poured a jug of milk over her. Within a few hours she too died, faithfully attended by a doll on each arm. There was the little boy in Blackball who ran out in the storm and fell in the raging channel at the side of the main road and whose body was found an hour later pulped on the rocks at the foot of a waterfall; and the fair-haired little girl spread-eagled in all the grotesqueness of death behind the bloodstained car.

Our visitors were frequent. My parents came for a happy month. At Stillwater I drove my car along the railway-tracks (officially approved) and my mother was lifted straight from carriage to car. A frequent visitor was my father-in-law, T. C. Brash, then executive officer of the Dairy Board. It was old territory to him, he having been manager of the Totara Flat dairy factory at the age of twenty-two. He was the most amiable of men but I once deeply displeased him by investing seven pounds ten in a nebulous gold prospecting scheme in the Grey River, opposite Blackball. 'It wasn't much,' I pleaded; it was too much to throw away, he maintained. The prospecting led to the Argo Gold Company and when it closed two years later I had received seventy-five pounds in dividends. This represented one thousand per cent profit on the outlay, against which there is no argument.

Another occasional visitor to the surgery was Mr H. E. Holland, member for the district and leader of the Labour Party. He suffered from angina for which I prescribed on several occasions. I was once invited by him to travel in his birdcage from Stillwater to Christchurch. He was a gentle man, one of his party's pioneers, who tried to combine the humanities with politics.

Once (still talking of visitors) I came home one afternoon, worried over a very ill patient who, despite treatment which should have been successful, was getting worse. And there, at home, drinking tea with my wife was Dr George Home and his wife. Truly he was heaven sent. Once more I sat at his feet. The pus was draining freely, I said, but more was building up. Where? He told me where it was and what I should do. When he had gone I returned to the patient. I followed instructions. The pus gushed forth. 'Thank God,' said the patient.

At first there was no telephone. It came eventually in the form of a party line for nine. For the first few days it was an exciting public plaything with no thought of privacy. Whenever the doctor's call came through every phone was lifted. One woman rang me, 'Doctor, I think you should know that all that woman has been telling you is lies.'

On 17 June 1929, New Zealand from Auckland to the Bluff was rocked by the Murchison earthquake. Blackball, only sixty miles away and precariously poised on a plateau, not only rocked but wavered. I have written elsewhere, in an essay called 'The Day of the Earthquake', published in *Growl You May But Go You Must* (Wellington, Reed, 1968), of the local details, and need repeat few of them here. Blackball was territorially isolated. No one was killed, but forty-two miners were injured by falls of coal. For once, the disaster could not be attributed to the Blackball Coal Company. As my next door neighbour, Charlie Duske, a fervent unionist, said, 'The bloke what's done that is too strong for us'. Though almost every housewife had her kitchen floor covered with smashed crockery and bottles of preserves, and almost every house-holder's backyard was littered with bricks from his chimney while his tank, torn from its fittings, rolled back and forth in the wind, yet there was a pooling of effort in the recovery, a selection of priorities by a form of communal goodwill. We had none of the hazards of bureaucracy. My work was of course tremendously increased and my resources decreased. The shelves in the surgery, recently painted, were bare and on the floor were the fragments of nearly a hundred Winchesters and bottles, their contents swirling and fuming in a mammoth incompatibility. But some bottles of pills and crystals had survived including phenobarbitone, bromides and chloral hydrate. From these I made up large stock quantities as a substitute for the tranquillizers of today. This mixture became very popular. Children would arrive in the surgery:

'Please, Mum says could she have another bottle of the earthquake medicine?'

We were happy in Blackball. We did not have to pay for rent, rates, telephone, electricity or coal. I was trusted in a friendly community though of course was never above criticism. In return we tried to repay. I gave frequent courses on first aid, joined one of the Lodges and became chairman of their debating club which involved me annually in the Greymouth competitions. In our front room the W.E.A. box scheme, inaugurated by Professor Shelley and supervised by Mr J. Johnson of Christchurch, met fortnightly, with an enthusiastic cross-section of about twenty from teacher to trucker, studying literature, art, music and drama. At the back of the section was a large shed which my wife fitted out as a kindergarten and for which I made a dozen small tables and chairs. A Wellington friend who was an unemployed kindergarten teacher lived with us. The pupils paid her one shilling a week. The idea was new to Blackball but nothing sinister could be found and soon it was well-approved.

One day a comprehensive book catalogue arrived from Gordon and Gotch in Melbourne. I recklessly ticked off my choice. My wife added hers. Later the local carrier left two massive cases on the verandah. I wrote a cheque on a Greymouth bank and posted it to Melbourne. All so simple.

Living was cheap. I paid back all my debts including that to Professor Hewitson with whom I had an amusing correspondence, he demurring about taking anything and I insisting on compound interest, which neither of us could work out with confidence. At length we compromised and he paid the money into a fund for indigent students.

Blackball was a good setting both for the Depression and the precarious years of an early family. (We had three children before we left.) We were digging in. Ambition was to come later. Though grim and grimy (my daughter, on seeing her first snow: 'Mummy, mummy, come and see the white soot') it was washed by the rains and swept by the winds to a tolerable state. The salary was small but precious, the more so as it obviated any barrier of fee between patient and doctor. It was in the evenings that we savoured our satisfaction. The surgery was shut. No confinement was pending. The children were asleep. Before the blazing fire I read aloud to my wife while she continued knitting. Simple pleasures? Yes. Rich simple pleasures. Every morning the press told of the stress in the outside world. From various medical friends I learned of the hazards of private practice. We were confirmed in our intention to ride out the Depression in Blackball.

But no one in New Zealand could escape the Depression, which permeated the country and in due course came to Blackball. The sale of coal fell off. The mine went from three shifts to two and then one. Men dropping out were not replaced. Two small mines, Cascade and Charming Creek, went onto the co-operative system whereby owner and worker shared profits and losses. The other mines protested by token strikes against unionists setting up tents with the enemy. But any strike

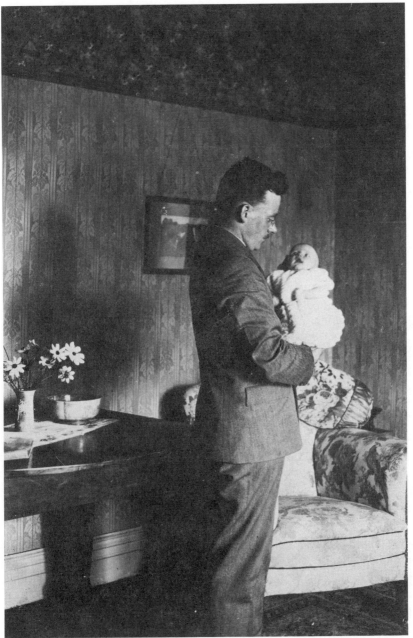

The author with his daughter Margaret, Blackball, 1928

was now only a symbol and no longer a weapon. At Blackball, interest shifted to an unexpected development by the Company. A new shaft was driven a mile or so from the main drive. The coal was to reach the bins by water propulsion and down an elaborate wooden flume. The Union approved. The new coal would be much more accessible and working conditions would be easier. A gang, selected by the mine manager on a basis that puzzled the rest, spent months on the preliminary work. When it was finished and the mining about to begin the secret had to come out.

The secret was that the workers on the flume represented a break-away group about to engage in co-operative mining. Their leader was W. Balderstone, late secretary of the Union. The Union's reaction was incredulity, followed by a blaze of hostility. The loyal miners, very much in the majority, heard the news on Saturday morning. A body of them set out to wreck the flume or to beat up any co-operatives. I stood at the door of the surgery and watched them, over a hundred, streaming up the hill. One called to me gaily, 'Get your stuff ready, Doc. The corpses will be down soon.'

But he was wrong. No co-operatives were about. Guarding the flume were some mine officials, several policemen, a few conservatives. The invaders began to argue and lost the initiative. They returned to the miners' hall to plan action. But the other side had foreseen all this. Before the end of the week there were fifty-five policemen in Blackball and most of them were there for many months. The flume was guarded day and night.

The Union of course immediately went on strike until the co-operatives were dismissed. It was a pathetic reprisal. The strike hurt no one but themselves. The Company announced that as the mine had always been run at a loss the strike would greatly improve the balance sheet.

Yet it was an ugly strike, lasting nine months. The strikers declared to the world the fervour of their industrial faith, but the world ignored it. The Christchurch papers printed nothing, the Greymouth papers only the minimum. The 1913 strike has become a fact of history but the 1931 strike, though bigger and more important, has been lost. The strikers did not qualify for the dole. Other miners could contribute sympathy only. The strikers went prospecting for gold and a few drifted away. Some doubled up with relatives or used any savings and in general lived miserably.

After the first clash a siege developed. The Company had great resources and time was on its side. The co-operatives, steadily producing coal and filling the orders, could be ostracized but not intimidated. The Union could not win. At the same time it could not bear to lose. It needed a nearer target.

Maintenance work in the mine and the generating plant which supplied the town with electricity were kept going by deputies and those who did not belong to the Union. When the Union ordered all its members out, two, the Levings, father and son, continued to work claiming they were members of the Engineers' Union. The Miners' Union refuted this and informed the management that the union would never work with scabs like the Levings.

The struggle intensified on this new aspect. Day and night the Levings' house was picketed by the miners and day and night guarded by the police. All through the night rocks and stones landed on the roof. The two went to work under police escort. Later, each walked through the jeering mob handcuffed to a constable. Then one morning the police swept them off in a car. The car set out the second morning and had four flat tyres in the first twenty yards. The daily walk was resumed. The enmity increased. It was directed against the Levings and not against the police who were good-natured and came largely from Auckland and were being treated to many new experiences, including snow. Hate by an individual can be dangerous but hate by a mob means violence. On one occasion the elder Leving, marching up the road handcuffed, was lined up in the sights of a man with a .303 rifle at a window. The pressure was being taken on the trigger when a constable walked in between and by a second a death was averted. Tradesmen refused to deliver goods. An alleged sympathizer had the verandah of his house wrecked by dynamite.

Then one morning the elder Leving did not go to work. It was not victory yet but the enemy was cracking for he strained his back and was unfit. This, the whole town knew, was a device to get signed on to compensation and retain his position without its rigours. But the town was confident this would not work. The doctor, their doctor, would never do anything so infamous as to put him on compensation even if his back were in several pieces.

So I had to go and see him, the crowd round the house passing me in cheerfully enough. I decided that the back injury though not severe was genuine but this was a minor matter. He was a wretched shaking mass of anxiety, on the verge of breakdown. His defiant front was a thin mask. I pleaded with him to give in. The fight was hopeless. Today, tomorrow, next week – he might survive till then but what about next year and the rest of his life? I proposed terms. I would put him on compensation for a few days. He would persuade his son to stay home and look after him. They would promise that they would never go back to the mine and I would undertake to stop all the hostile demonstrations. In the end he agreed, gratefully, I thought. I then found the president and secretary of the

Union. They were less pleased than I expected. They said bluntly that they did not trust the Levings. I said they had to and that he couldn't work even if he wanted to. On this assurance they stopped all demonstrations that night. Everyone slept, including myself.

The next morning there were two red hot items of news. One was that the Levings were back at work in the engine room and the other was that the doctor was a rat.

I lived it down eventually but not easily or happily. I was never called to the Levings again. The wearisome picketing began once more. Suddenly, representatives of the mine owners arrived from Wellington to discuss the matter of reopening the mine. Although the miners wanted to work desperately they still laid out some stiff demands. To them all, the company agreed. Part of the agreement was that the Levings should be dismissed and never again be employed by the Blackball Coal Co. The economic loss was an ideological victory. The matter was concluded in the miners' hall one midday. I was coming up the main road having just finished a confinement and the street was almost blocked with shouting cheering men. I sought out the Union secretary, Mountford, and told him he had a fine new son. His elation continued but I like to think it now had a parental component. Anyhow he called the boy Victor.

So work resumed. There were now two hostile unions working their respective mines. But there was only one Medical Association, which had expelled the co-operatives. The latter were now my private patients. But I did not – in fact could not – charge them. Their co-operative mine was not yet paying. I have no skill in getting blood from a stone. So for a time I treated them free. This placed me at the very hub of the industrial struggle. The Association reduced my salary. This was in keeping with the times and also because the reserves were becoming depleted. The co-operatives gave me a small grant. This meant that I was caught in the crossfire between two masters. It was obviously a system that could not last.

The industrial hatred intensified. Each group went to its own pub. The co-operatives were not allowed into the miners' hall even for pictures. They would not sit together in my waiting room. They wanted separate surgery hours which I refused. They bought their own drugs and I mixed them without compunction. It was even suggested that they build their own surgery. In fact before long everything was black or white except the surgery which remained a kind of drab grey. Eventually I was instructed by the Association that I was not to treat the co-operatives.

I pretended not to have understood. I drew imaginary pictures of the consequences. If a co-operative went beserk and was a danger to members of the Association, could I be permitted to quieten him with a sedative? If an enemy fell in the street, could I help him to his feet? If a miner stabbed a co-operative could I, a bystander, intervene and stop the haemorrhage and so limit the charge to one of assault and not murder?

My levity and my imagination failed. I was informed that my position, my surgery and my drugs belonged to the Association. I would have to respect their wishes. These were that I must cease attendances of any sort on the 'Balderstone crowd'.

It was an incredible position. Even in warfare the medical services of one side are available to the other. There had been much sympathy for the Association till then, but now round the countryside, in Paparoa, in Greymouth, this was replaced by outspoken criticism. Professor Hercus wrote from Dunedin for the truth about the rumours he had heard. Then a majority of the executive waited on me to inform me I was not carrying out their wishes. I said I was bound by professional and humanitarian obligations which had nothing to do with their wishes. I had always treated everybody. I always would. They nodded and went away as if they were not surprised. A little later I was asked to attend a full meeting of the executive. My own private grapevine informed me that this was the showdown. And it was. They were quite blunt. They wanted my promise that I would never treat any of the other group or any of their dependants at any time in the future no matter what the malady or the circumstances.

This was as far as negotiation could go. I think they were a little surprised at the vigour of my refusal. I left no room for compromise. I said that from the time of Christ my profession had regarded all sick as equals. To change this was beyond the power of any dissidents from Blackball. I had my resignation written out. I flicked it down the table to the secretary and walked out.

My sacrifice in this was less than might appear. Dr Ray of Greymouth was to go to England for a year and we had arranged that I was to be his locum at a suitable time. I now suggested starting in three months and he agreed.

So the Blackball adventure ended on a sour note but it could have been worse. All parties were, I think, sad about the conflict of ideologies. Our differences were not personal. They kept saying in the Association, 'Now we'll get someone who'll do what he's told,' but this was mere bravado. Both mines gave me a farewell and a presentation – vases from Paparoa and a small bottle of gold dust from Blackball. Everyone tried to be hearty and few succeeded. The only one to come out of it with credit was Hippocrates.

They got another doctor, an elderly man who for many reasons was an unfortunate choice. He died a few years later in the Greymouth old men's home. The prohibition on his treating co-operatives ceased to have much point for he soon was hardly treating anyone. Many Blackball patients came to Greymouth to Dr Bird or to me. Only in Blackball did the factions persist. Once, twenty-five years later, two women arrived in my waiting room in Christchurch. They sat rigidly staring at the opposite wall, pretending the other was not there, all in loyalty to a cause they had probably now forgotten. There was less industrial purity about Balderstone who about the same time consulted me and on behalf of his group later sent me a truck of coal.

There are now few survivors of those contestants. The mines are flooded and the only sound is when a stone rattles noisily down the cliff face. The station has closed, the bridge has gone and there is no doctor now in Blackball. The air is clean again, the bush-scented air of the Coast. The old issues have been swept away by government intervention. No history books nor encyclopedias refer to the strike. In Parliament Mr Holland asked when the Blackball mine (on a Crown lease) was going to resume, and the minister said that the mine was freehold and he did not know. The annual report to Parliament from the Mines Department does not mention the strike. There is no reference to it in the Appendices to the Journals. It not only failed to make history, it failed to make news. The brave play had been staged but the auditorium was empty. They had exploited aggression and had been counter-attacked with indifference.

I have been back, thirty years later. The town is cleaner, smaller and duller. The surgery has gone. The house is deserted, the doors flapping. At the corner between the store and the pub where on Saturday nights they would mill and shout, argue and drink, all is now quiet. I saw a pretty girl in a new car elegantly sweep round the corner. I came away. It was alien territory. It belonged by right of occupation to declamatory miners vigorously pursuing the adventures of their lives.

I was a year in Greymouth, a precious year among medical colleagues again. The senior member was Dr McBrearty with whom, as Dr Ray's locum, I was in partnership. He, like his father, was the esteemed 'Dr Jim' of Greymouth. He died during my term there. The leader in our medical world was Dr C. Moore, Superintendent of the hospital, an extraordinary man who worked hard and played hard, and accepted any challenge of medicine, pediatrics, surgery, orthopaedics, obstetrics, or psychiatry. He organized for us regular clinical meetings at the hospital. Dr Bird and I did the general practice of the town. Greymouth has been extremely well served by its permanent doctors. Both Dr Jims, the late Dr Bird and the present Dr Ray have spent their whole careers in Greymouth and all have been tireless workers. Dr Wilkinson, later Superintendent at Hanmer, was at Wallsend and Dr Meade at Runanga. Dr Wilson, my fellow house surgeon at New Plymouth, was now surgeon at Hokitika. In the hospital was the assistant superintendent, Dr Bell, brother of Dr Muriel Bell, and the house surgeon Dr Russell Fraser, now professor of endocrinology at Hammersmith post-graduate hospital. With the exception of Dr Meade we were all graduates from Otago and were all under forty. We formed a keen and harmonious group.

But it was a year of unremitting work. Dr Ray, able and energetic, had left me a very large practice. To this was added many of my old patients from Blackball and the Grey Valley. Rarely did I have more than two meals a day, a rushed breakfast and a more leisurely hot dinner in the late evening. There was much midwifery and I went on collecting samples of blood. One woman escaped by stating that she was glad she had come to me instead of another doctor she had heard of, who always stuck needles in all his patients.

Any doctor on the Coast has to be versatile. As honorary medical officer of the boxing club I once passed a boxer as fit and then attended him when he collapsed in the ring. As honorary physician I received him into one of my hospital beds and gave the anaesthetic when Dr Moore trephined his skull. He died and as police medical officer I did the post-mortem and gave evidence at the inquest.

I attended one day a man of fifty-three for an acute medical condition and noted that he had a badly withered leg. It was due, he said, to a stroke at the age of three. Dr Jim had said so. He added that he had got off 'better than the other kids'. He referred me to his mother for details. She was an active octogenarian who confirmed an epidemic of strokes fifty years before, involving eleven children in two streets in the course of a few weeks. She gave me some names and I managed to trace two of them. They had the typical lesions of poliomyelitis.

This epidemic must have been in 1880. It was before the first recorded epidemic in New Zealand and may well have been the first in the country. Poliomyelitis was not diagnosed even in America till 1894. In Greymouth at the time there were probably over one thousand children. If eleven were paralysed about one hundred were also infected without paralysis. What about the other ninety per cent? There was no isolation, no precautions, no inoculation, no treatment. About seventy-five years later the Royal Australasian College of Physicians at a Wellington conference advised the government that the rigid isolation which was closing schools was unnecessary. Greymouth could have confirmed the decision.

Occasionally on a Saturday there was a cabaret or a picture show. I saw my first 'talkie' in Greymouth: 'A Cuckoo in the Nest' with Ralph Lynne, Tom Walls and Robertson Hare. I thought at the time that no higher standard in entertainment could ever be reached. I even stayed awake all through.

Towards the end of the year there came an adventurous weekend. I went to Christchurch where an agent (father of Sir Charles Hercus) waylaid me, urging me to buy the house and practice of Dr William Irving at 56 Armagh St. I went through the house, curiously, enviously, but vainly as one might gaze in a jeweller's window. I had little money, and less of the confidence that was essential for a city practice. Two other country districts had recently invited me to initiate a practice. To this the agent said, 'Well, you might do better in that place in Southland'. This suggestion that I could not measure up to a city annoyed me. I went through it again with my wife. She was concerned only with the house. 'It would be fun,' she said, imagining each child with a bedroom and a private rumpus room. 'But impossible. Think of the rates, the painting, the upkeep.' This also annoyed me. She was implying that because we were poor we always would be. I took my father over it. 'The value is there,' he agreed, thinking of a quarter acre in the heart of Christchurch. 'But you can't find the deposit and I'm afraid I can't help you.' I knew this as I had recently been helping him. I then got in touch with my father-in-law. What did he think and would he back me? He had one answer to all this. Buy.

So I bought – as I had intended to do, from the beginning. Christchurch was my home; here were my parents in the same street, my three brothers, my friends and my colleagues of Medical School days. I knew I was to be permanently in Christchurch. Canterbury was my place.

After that it was all anticipation. We drove back arguing as to how many bedrooms there were on the top floor (actually six). We passed the Riccarton Hotel a few hours after the proprietor (Donald Fraser) had been shot by cartridges purchased, according to the police, on the West Coast. I was congratulated by Drs Moore and Bird on my clever escape. The next day the police summoned me to the station. As police surgeon I expected to be confronted with a corpse. Instead I was informed that Christchurch had installed its first traffic lights at the intersection of Colombo and Cashel Streets and that I had driven through when the light was red. I wrote a contrite letter and the light suddenly went green again.

In the closing stages, my Greymouth colleagues treated me to a farewell party in one of the hotels. It was a typical West Coast party where the occasion is remembered better than the details. They presented me with a leather medical bag which I still carry in the locked boot of my car.

So we came to Christchurch, my wife and I, three children, a truckload of furniture, an inflexible mortgage and some precious notebooks recording blood counts.

154

8

Pilgrimage to Christchurch

Christchurch was home. Appropriately, the first house I ever owned was in Christchurch. It was a massive construction of kauri and totara designed round gracious and expensive living. Upstairs there were six bedrooms in a row. The two unadorned rooms were for maids. The other four had open fireplaces. By each fireplace was an elaborate porcelain and brass handle which, when turned through half a circle, would ring the appropriate bell in the kitchen and so summon the maid. They were all in perfect working order except for the maid. There were additions such as a boxroom, a dressing room, a coal shed, a servery and three reception rooms.

Outside the house were other additions: a croquet green, an outside toilet obviously for the domestic staff, a tool-shed, an artesian well and a detached building of three rooms, one of which was a carpenter's workshop. It had a splendid bench and vice. I, whose previous work-shops had been improvised from a couple of fruit cases on some back verandah, found this a persistent lure. It undoubtedly shortened the presale hesitation.

It was a house of charm and dignity, a house for mistress and maids, a house built round the conventions of society and an established order, a house rapidly stepping back into social history. It was, so many people must have said, the wrong house for me. What they really meant was that I was the wrong person for that house. In this they erred. My wife and I had no longing for a gentleman's residence. We were too close to the soil of New Zealand for that. But we saw in it a great potential for a family home, and that is what it became, by the simple integration of its inhabitants. Each child had his or her bedroom, grew up there, moved out, brought back their own children and never ceased to regard it as home. It had that rare asset of the modern day, space; and as a result it had hundreds of visitors and dozens of guests. At first the croquet green at the back would be possessed on fair afternoons by nuggety little thugs on loan from various kindergartens. Then the tradition carried on through primary and secondary schools and university. In the university phase we were almost dispossessed; I would come home from a late call and find the kitchen full of noise, steam and odours. There would be a dozen of them plying knives, forks and tongues, with a frying-pan bubbling and the zip steaming. They would give me the cool stare due to an intruding stranger, and would go on eating my eggs and bacon.

There was an occasion when Christchurch accommodated a conference of international philosophers. One evening was devoted to a party at my house arranged by my son. It was essential, he insisted, that I put in an appearance and breathe some words of welcome. So I let him lead me to one group of half a dozen or so. 'That was a fine paper your brother gave this afternoon' said one. 'But did you agree with it?' Gently I explained that my brother was my son and that I hadn't heard it and in any case would not have understood it. 'I am not a philosopher,' I said positively. He turned his back on me and addressed the others, 'How would he know he is not a philosopher?' Immediately they all began speaking. I drifted off, duty done. I never knew the outcome. I knew I was not a philosopher for the same reason that I knew that I was not a budgie or a porcupine. I sometimes envy the mental gymnastics of the philosophers and their invariable ability to land safely on both feet.

I still have the house and as a symbol of family integration the light still falls on it. Each in his own room had a precious and private freedom and did not surrender it prematurely. There might be a certain freedom in a flat in the big world but it was a poor substitute for freedom in a personal world. Fill the house as you might: it was never crowded. Here at times have stayed many of our friends and most of our relations. But there have been others: elderly women in transit, distressed girls, once seven stranded ballet dancers, two Gilbert Islanders studying at Canterbury Training College, undergraduates, another time an overflow from Bishop Julius hostel, refugees from Hitler's Europe. Here the Christchurch branch of the Home Science Alumnae was formed. I recall musical and poetry evenings, two weddings and a golden wedding, billiard parties, committee meetings of the S.C.M., of the Sunshine League, of the B.M.A. The back door was always open.

The Christchurch medical world in 1933 was an untidy area. Specialization in neurology, orthopaedics, gynaecology, nephrology and cardiology, was only just beginning and its exponents still relied on general practice. There was no zoning, no partnerships, no private laboratories or radiology, no government subsidy, no medico-social workers. Appointments to the part-time hospital staff were honorary. Every doctor treated what came his way. General practitioners did surgery if the case were straightforward and the fee fairly certain. It was considered unethical to charge doctors and their families, ministers and their families, nurses and the destitute. Half the doctors had Lodge lists (one pound a year for a family of four). The main private hospitals were Calvary (then Lewisham), St George's and The Limes (now the site of the Town Hall). Essex and Lyndhurst were the only large obstetric hospitals. There were many smaller private homes in the suburbs. In the previous decade the majority of the country districts had maternity hospitals built by the North Canterbury Hospital Board. Puerperal sepsis was common and domiciliary obstetrics was losing favour. There was a high incidence of scarlet fever. In the sanatorium were over three hundred cases of tuberculosis and a constant call for more beds. There were none of the modern outpatient clinics nor any building to house them.

There was also the deepening Depression. The press was disposed to ignore it. Sporting, racing, social chit-chat, entertainment, photos of local events filled a large portion of each issue. The Depression was ugly and not newsworthy. If ignored it might go away. The press gave more space to land sales, share markets, life insurance, retail bargains. But the undercurrents were deep. Christchurch was the only city where rioting did not occur. Of this period W. H. Scotter, in *A History of Canterbury, Vol. III: 1876-1950* (Christchurch, Whitcombe and Tombs, 1965), says:

> By 1933 many workers were at the end of their resources: according to D. G. Sullivan five thousand people were 'deep in poverty'. Relief helpers constantly came on families who had been living only on frosted tomatoes and potatoes, families who were almost destitute of clothing, firing, furniture and crockery. There were hundreds of homes where the bedclothes consisted of two grey blankets of a Government issue, supplemented by sacks when available. Mothers were known to feed their babies on sweetened water and a little biscuit; men working on the roads in sandshoes or boots without soles took no lunch so that those at home should not be deprived. Children could not attend school because they did not have enough clothes.

On this stony ground I pitched my tent. The children went on being excited. I went on being apprehensive. Dr Irving introduced me to twelve patients, half of whom I never saw again. This was a revival of the Te Aroha fiasco, paying for a practice which did not exist. In both cases I had purchased a solid right to participate in the Depression.

I did all the right things: put ethically faultless notices in the papers, called on my seniors and was kindly received, and was given a few anaesthetics by some of the surgeons; revived, less formally, old friendships with the younger doctors, flicked the red light on at my gate every evening and an hour later flicked it off. Only the moths came.

In lieu of patients I called on some relatives including my great-hearted aunt, then bedridden. She predicted my success, knowing nothing about it, and then cross-examined me as to my hours, telephone number, degrees, specialities . . . . This was all idle enough till I saw her niece noting it all down. I in turn cross-examined. What were they up to? My alarm grew and eventually I forced out of them the whole incredible story. They had arranged with a jobbing printer for two thousand cards advertising and recommending me with no more subtlety than if I were a brand of coffee. The girls were then going round on Saturday afternoon to slip a card under the front door of the best houses in Cashmere and Fendalton. I left them in tears. The horror of the whole thing was the ease with which it might have succeeded. I could imagine at the next B.M.A. meeting half a dozen members calling the chairman's attention to a certain card . . . and I protesting against their disbelief that I knew nothing about it.

It came as a miserable truth that the medical profession was also a victim of the Depression. As I went on my visits, in Harley most waiting-rooms were empty. The secretary of the Canterbury Division sat at his desk at three p.m., head back, mouth agape, noisily snoring. 'Well, I'll have to go old man. Got an appointment. Can't miss ten and six you know.' I went on trying to swim upstream in the rapids. Mentally I joined the sullen group of unemployed who filled all the seats in the Square. There was one desperate fortnight when, as in Te Aroha, I did not see a single patient.

To cover the misery of that period I got out my blood counts again. They were interesting but baffling. I wanted help. There was no medical library in the hospital. Instead there was that large-hearted gentleman, Dr A. B. Pearson, the pathologist. He advised me and sent me home with large numbers of his own American medical journals. Even though I might have to finish it in a debtors' prison I now had the material for an M.D. thesis. About the same time the Hunterian Society in England announced the subject of its annual essay, 'Midwifery in General Practice', which to me meant midwifery in Blackball. It was open to all doctors in the Empire but had never previously been won outside Britain. I rejected (repeatedly) the absurdity of competing, but the idea would not go away. It was compounded of the years of silent reading at Fairview, the hours of silent waiting through the second stage of labour at Blackball and the silent days of unemployment in Christchurch.

As always, the tragedy had to be ruffled by the comedy. A letter one Friday informed me that a sum of money was waiting my collection at the Public Trust. The office had shut before I got there and over the week-end my wife and I had built it up into a prodigious sum left by some grateful patient. Monday morning revealed that the grateful patient was a debt collector in Greymouth, who unable to meet my account, had insisted on the names and addresses of some of my worst bad debts. Later he died and his papers revealed that he had collected five shillings on my account. This, less tax, commission and administration costs, left a residue of about two and sixpence for which I duly signed.

Dr Irving, though he was vice-president of the N.Z. Obstetricians and Gynaecologists Society, had only one midwifery case booked. He presented her to me as if she were something special from Kimberly. She was an elderly primapara. Before she could make her first antenatal visit she wrote and said that 'all things considered' she thought it would be preferable for her to be attended by the specialist, Dr Mark Brown. He was a friend of mine and it was natural, when his bout of influenza coincided with the onset of her labour, that he should ask me to deputize for him. She was in much distress and welcomed me warmly. Everything went well. We became good friends and she was my patient for years.

I was busy at my blood counts one morning when I received a ring from Dr Wm. Bates, an elderly practitioner. I knew him slightly and was a little surprised and more than a little gratified that he had heard of me. Was I free, he asked? Could I see a case with him? A difficult one, rather urgent? He gave a number in Ferry Road. He was there now. He would wait.

I ran downstairs. My wife called from the washhouse, 'What is it? Got a case?'

'Case? I've got a consultation.'

'Hooray.'

'Hooray,' I echoed slamming the car door.

I found the address. Dr Bates was standing at the gate. I pulled up and crossed to him with what I imagined was the confident smile of a consultant. He regarded me warily.

'Do you want to see me?' he asked. I explained that he had just sent for me. Suddenly his face softened in comprehension.

'I must have rung the wrong number. It was Dr L. A. Bennett I wanted, the surgeon. You're not a surgeon are you? You must be this young chap that's just started. Well, fancy that – fancy my ringing the wrong number.'

He seemed to think it very funny. We shared the joke together, he getting the lion's share. His patient had no phone. He asked me to ring 'the right Dr Bennett' at the telephone-box at the corner. This I did. As I arrived home my wife said, 'Well that didn't take you long.' In her voice was an undertone of admiration. 'No. There wasn't much to it. We decided to hand it over to a surgeon.' It was my first consultation in Christchurch. The fees amounted to a debit of one penny.

Not far away was the hospital, the land of promise for the ambitious. I would walk in boldly twice a month to medical meetings and tip-toe in cautiously at other times to see an occasional patient. Here in the distance I would sometimes glimpse the benign dictator of the hospital, Dr Walter Fox. He had surprised me when I first came to Christchurch by calling on me before I could call on him. He sat on the edge of my couch with his hands cupped over his silver topped walking stick and fired questions at me. It had a grim resemblance to an oral examination. He assured me that every doctor who came to Christchurch had made a living. But he did not explain how.

I progressed at a snail's pace. Several patients with friends on the Coast booked confinements, but the payment of the fee was far away. A few strangers appeared in the waiting room, mainly casuals drifting in off the street, bemusedly taking my advice and forgetting about the fee. No solid heart to a practice there. A new Lodge was formed in a government institution and I happily agreed to be the Medical Officer. I did a locum for Dr Stevens of New Brighton.

Despite all this I could not meet the first mortgage payment. My fault without doubt, implied the lawyers at a bitter meeting. They tried to encourage me to greater effort by raising the rate of interest.

One melancholy evening was filled with the mathematics of my economics. The future expenditure was predictable and the graph could be drawn. But the graph of income alongside it? Draw it as optimistically as possible yet never the twain could meet.

The next morning Dr Fox rang. He wished to see me at the hospital at ten a.m. In his office he elaborated. Dr Duncan, medical officer for Charitable Aid, was going on an extended visit to England. A replacement was needed. Also a medical officer was required for the Jubilee Home (female geriatric hospital). If I would do this he had other work in the hospital for me – he outlined something like duties of a medical registrar, though one task was lecturing to nurses in surgery. ('Pardon me, Dr Fox. I presume you mean medicine.' 'I did not. I said surgery and I meant surgery.') He would like me in from nine a.m. till midday, five days a week. Salary six hundred and fifty pounds a year. Was I interested?

I suppose I nodded for I would not have trusted myself to speak. He was not deceived. He immediately went into details. I remember, 'And if you want a diagnosis ask the porters. They know everything.' He finished up with, 'Start tomorrow. Nine o'clock.'

The money meant that every day earned me almost two pounds. The modern doctor would be amused. But a house surgeon at that time would take thirteen years to earn my salary. A man on the dole (ten shillings a week) would take twice as long. It bent one of my graphs at a delirious angle. Now, over forty years later, I have been (and still am) employed by the North Canterbury Hospital Board in a variety of services, all continuous except for the war years.

The other benefits of the appointment were hardly less than the money. I was in the hospital every day making fresh acquaintances, listening, learning, conforming. I gave lectures in surgery and in the process taught myself more surgery than I ever taught my nurses. Jubilee Home was an austere place run with such economy that it lacked light, colour and animation. It was permeated by the odour of unwashed linen. It is now totally reformed. In the thirties the new specialty of geriatrics had not arrived. Bottle Lake Hospital was almost entirely reserved for scarlet fevers (three hundred and sixty seven cases that year). I conformed to the bad standard of treatment. We insisted on extravagances of isolation and on an irrational period of convalescence (four weeks for adults and six weeks for children). I began to visit my Charitable Aid cases (this phrase was not an ugly one). As expected, they were of all types: the proud and the independent, the helpless who lacked initiative, and the dissolute types – inevitable burdens of society in any community. The great majority were worthy folk, baffled by the times but co-operative and grateful. It was easy to establish good relations with them, particularly as there was no money bar. There were times when I could have been back in Blackball.

Another involvement with the unemployed was the examination of married men selected for labour camps in the country. Their only escape was to plead medical unfitness and to have it proved by a medical examination at hospital. Gladly Dr Fox handed this over to me and at the end of each morning I would deal with up to a dozen despondent men sitting on long forms in Outpatients. If they were passed they went into the country, lived in tin shacks, paid for blankets, worked in water with no drying facilities and got thirty to thirty-five shillings a week to support themselves and their families in town.

Were they physically fit for this? Perhaps. Were they fit psychologically to desert wife, home and family, in the crisis of destitution, at the very time when male support was most needed? No, they were not. In all of them was either the anxiety neurosis or its potential. The great majority were certified by me as unfit. Dr Fox fully approved. So probably did many of my colleagues in other centres, for after a while married men were no longer sent to camp. One of the causes of rioting was thus removed.

Just as medical knowledge has advanced enormously in the last fifty years so has the doctor-patient relationship. Fifty years ago each individual doctor had his loyal contingent, but the profession as a whole lacked a good image. It had vast authority which is never a popular commodity. It presided officially over occasions of public health, medical jurisprudence and death. Medical services were regarded by the public as transactions in which a fee was paid for a service performed. If that service was merely an opinion that no treatment was feasible then the fee was resented. Doctor and patient looked at the matter each from his own angle but the fee always tended to widen the gap.

Today, how different. The patient is better educated, more tolerant, more co-operative. The doctor now has much more to offer, effective treatments having replaced the empiricisms and the placebos. The humanities have now moved into his therapeutic field and the fear of the fee has dimmed. Money is now more plentiful and less exalted. The government bears much of the burden, and inevitably under the compulsion of social evolution will, in the future, bear it all. The public now judges the profession itself, and finds little of difference between doctor and doctor. The setting invites discussion between patient and doctor, not bargaining.

I was once consulted by a legal gentleman, elderly, conservative, inflexible, in my surgery. He laid his stick, hat and gloves on the table, composed himself in a chair and then divulged the purpose of his visit, which was to inform me that in the future I was to replace his present doctor. I asked who had been his doctor. He said that we each belonged to a profession where confidences were respected. Despite the increasing restlessness in the waiting room and the constant ringing of the bell, he stayed for fifteen minutes. I felt I should have offered him a whisky. Three months later he was back and he stormed into the surgery, almost incoherent with rage. He had been kept waiting six minutes for his appointment. An appointment was an appointment and was sacred. He banged the table with his stick. I had miners bang the table in Blackball but their grievance was against the capitalists. I waved olive branches. They might as well have been burning brands. Whatever his malady was he took it with him making it quite clear that our association was finished. It was probably our sole point in common. Any consultation with him (or anyone else) could be interrupted by a peremptory summons to a confinement. A foetus, impatient to see the waiting world, has little respect for the legal profession. Poor man. He is now long dead but in his day, for reasons he never understood, he doggedly kept the step in the Victorian march. At the present day the waiting patient waits; or tries another doctor. He does not storm. He is aware, as they were in Blackball, that only urgency determines medical priorities.

But in the old days when doctors were either good or bad they could easily become very good or very bad. They were the innocent victims of gossip, of repetitive, persistent, uninformed gossip, snowballing blindly along. Sometimes the core of such a panegyric was merit; more often it was the egotism that pretended the special knowledge. There are famous doctors today, particularly among the specialities. Their reputations are more soundly based on merit and are acknowledged by their colleagues who advertise them by referring patients to them. They no longer need to rely on the bubble of reputation.

In the middle thirties I became involved in such a process of public approbation. My midwifery practice began to increase. . . and increase. . . and increase. I built another room onto the surgery. It was soon inadequate. I was competing – with some embarrassment – with better obstetricians who had higher degrees and who had trained at the Rotunda or the great hospitals of England. I had trained on a solo course in Blackball.

Undoubtedly some of the public favour was due to my genuine interest in the subject. The miracle of birth had never ceased to fascinate me. At birth the physiology suddenly changes, smoothly and effectively, by a mechanism unknown. There is no experimental stage, no trial period, merely a confident start on a course of many decades. There are some scientists who claim that the whole biological world is born of trial and error, and its infinite varieties have been set up by chance. It is not a theory favoured by most obstetricians as they watch the miracle of a foetus adapting itself from one world to another in a few smooth minutes.

Before the beginning of the war I was granted the status of obstetric specialist. It had to be applied for and the outcome hung on how convincing was the letter of application. I quoted that I was on the staffs of St Helens and Karitane Hospitals, was superintendent of the newly formed obstetric wing at Calvary Hospital, editor of the O. & G. section of the *New Zealand Medical Journal*, medical officer for obstetrical research, vice-president of the N.Z. O. & G. Society and on the practical side had conducted approximately two thousand confinements with no maternal loss. It was perhaps a persuasive application but it would have failed today where the pre-requisites are more rigidly defined. When Lewisham Hospital began obstetrics it became a B grade training school for midwives, who had to be instructed by a medical superintendent approved by the department. Lecturing to the Sisters was a pleasant task, such was their sincerity and concentration. All who were available including the Reverend Mother took the course and at the end of the year all qualified. At the same time I became adviser to Calvary Hospital. It was an empty title. It was made plain by those who appointed me that my religion was wrong, my hospital experience was poor but that the first year of war had depleted the field. I was never asked for any advice and once, when I offered it, it was rejected.

Being a specialist was also an empty honour. It allowed one to charge a fee additional to the five pounds given by the government. I found this hard to do. Why should a patient whom I had attended twice before suddenly be charged extra for the same service just because I had written a letter to the Health Department? Yet I had to charge something. To entice patients with specialist services and general practitioner fees would not be ethical. So I did the best I could, not always successfully.

A married couple, apparently middle-aged, once consulted me. She was timid, drooping and colourless. He was granite-faced and aggressive. Before he entrusted his pregnant wife to me he wanted an agreement about fees. How much extra did I charge? It depended, I said. . . but he interrupted. It didn't depend. How much extra did I charge? On an impulse I said 'Two guineas'. He looked at me incredulously. 'Did you say two guineas?' Yes, I had said two guineas, now wishing I had said four. He got to his feet and jerked his wife up. 'Come, my dear, we will get our medical requirements elsewhere.' At the door he turned and said witheringly, 'We are not millionaires, you know.' I pictured him as a small retailer, shopping around. The contract would probably have been made if the fee had been one pound ninteen and eleven pence halfpenny.

Obstetrics predominated but was by no means exclusive. I was on the Honorary Staff of the hospital first as anaesthetist and then as assistant physician, went to innumerable meetings, became involved with Mr W. M. Cotter and Mr D. McK. Dickson in the first attempts at post-graduate education in Christchurch, was secretary of the Canterbury Division of the B.M.A. and of the now defunct Medical Club.

The M.D. thesis had gone in. I went to Dunedin and sat the examination which I found rather like the curate's egg. Before the examiners could come to grips with it the English examiners recommended that I be granted the degree with honours on the thesis alone. (This has been referred to by some of my friends as getting an M.D. by correspondence.)

The result of the Hunterian Society Essay confirmed that Blackball was part of the British Empire despite what the Miners' Union might think. The Secretary of the Society, Arthur Porritt, sent personal congratulations to a fellow student. Two circumstances of the presentation at the B.M.A. conference in Wellington gave me much pleasure. The proceedings were broadcast and listening in were my parents, my most sturdy supporters in the bad old days. And at the foot of the stairs of the Art Gallery Dr George Home was waiting with his wry smile and his head on one side, and almost certainly with an appropriate Gilbert and Sullivan quotation ready. Instead he put out his hand, saying 'Well, show me the bauble'.

Later I became (by examination) a Member of the Royal Australasian College of Physicians and subsequently a Fellow. I was the only candidate under the searchlights of three examiners. My most pleasant memory of that occasion is that it was due to me that the College once had one hundred per cent of passes.

Enough. This record might appear egotistic but emphatically is not. Egotism is to me abhorrent. It is also impossible with a medical school record like mine. This is a story not of me but of my times. I have listed some facts which are essential to the narrative. I know no way of telling them and at the same time dissociating myself.

The late thirties and the early forties were turbulent times in medical administration. For the first time the Government intervened. The intrusion was strongly resented and vigorously opposed. In the House, Savage said:

> I want our people to have security. I want to see humanity secured against poverty, secure in illness or old age.

The profession approved of this but not of the suggested methods. It claimed, quite rightly, that the practice of medicine involved delicate patient-doctor relationships that could never be covered by an Act of Parliament. It mistrusted Savage's ideal, suspecting that it was a smokescreen to hide the introduction of socialism. This socialism to us was a vague force aimed first at domination of the medical profession, then of the legal profession, and later of dentistry and the other professions.

It was a silly contention yet we firmly believed it. I spoke and wrote in vigorous support, putting forth views that I have long since abandoned. The Government seemed to think it was all a matter of money and kept raising the bid for a salaried service on a capitation scheme. Its progressive members such as D. G. McMillan and A. H. Nordmeyer went too fast. The profession had a resistance committee led by Dr P. S. Jameson who went too slowly. He was a magnificent warrior in a rearguard action but neither party was, in the early stages at least, prepared to yield enough to effect any compromise. And yet in the end the Government won. It agreed to a partial fee with a state subsidy. The subsidy has gone on increasing in range and amount. There is still the right to charge a private fee 'commensurate with the services given'. Patient and doctor often disagree about this as the doctor disagrees with his plumber and electrician who use the same method.

The present system of subsidized fees hangs on nothing but

compromise and lacks social stability. When, as president of the Canterbury Division of the B.M.A. (1956), I selected as the theme of my inaugural address the inevitability of the salaried state service, my audience was kindly but was not impressed. 'Not in our time, old man, I hope.' But the reasons for this prophecy (too lengthy to detail here) have not altered and the prediction persists as one item of a personal benign prophecy.

This was the period when obstetrics came out into the light. Previously it had been merely an appendage to general practice. Our instructors in Dunedin (Drs Riley, Ritchie and North) though excellent, were lecturers only and also general practitioners. All centres had their prominent obstetricians; Christchurch: Averill, Mark Brown, Ramsay, Jennings, Hartnell, Hunter, McMillan; Wellington: Ian Ewart and T. H. Corkill; Auckland: G. Levy and Paterson; Stratford: Dr Doris Gordon.

Of these the most spectacular was Dr Doris Gordon. This extraordinary person may have trailed the others in clinical knowledge but she led them in raising the status of obstetrics. Her first objective was to appoint a fulltime professor of obstetrics and gynaecology in the Medical School. She campaigned throughout New Zealand, aiming particularly at the wives of wealthy landowners. This ensured large cheques from the husbands. The cause was recognized as a good feminist one even if its object might be obscure. (Old lady at a bridge party: 'I've just put something in for this obstetrical chair but I have no idea what I would do with it if I got it.') Her campaign was successful. The salary of a professor was guaranteed and the inaugural professor was Sir Bernard Dawson, who was soon solidly established in the medical curriculum.

Having revitalized undergraduate teaching she now turned to post-graduate teaching. Her idea was to establish a centre in Auckland. She called an inaugural meeting in Wellington with representatives from Treasury, the Health Department, the B.M.A. and the O. & G. Society. She made an impassioned plea for the new hospital and she carried most of her audience with her. I was the only one who spoke vigorously against it. It was wartime. That morning we had heard of the first engagement of New Zealand troops in the western desert and I at least could imagine gaping wounds, blood, flies, sand and thirst. The country was desperately short of building materials and labour. England was starving for the foodstuffs of New Zealand. Any distraction from the national effort for survival must have a valid necessity. In times of war men think of the defences and women think of the defenders. At the luncheon recess Dr Gordon came up to me:

'You're not well,' she informed me. 'Obviously you're not well. You've been overworking. You should pack up and have a long holiday.'

In the end each of us was successful. The war was won and the women's hospital in Auckland was built – but not till after the war.

She and I were closely associated in obstetrical matters. She came to Christchurch and addressed the O. & G. Society. I went to Stratford and addressed the Taranaki Division, where in 1926 I had attended the inaugural meeting. She once wrote a lengthy denunciation of the abortionist and sent it to me for literary criticism. I thought it was awful and wrote and said so. She then appeared guest-like on my doorstep and was taken in. All the spare time of the next week was spent in literary conference. It was a hopeless collaboration. She amended the text behind my back. I did the same to her. Eventually we sent it to Professor Dawson. It came back, reduced to half and red-pencilled on every page. It next went to the advertising firm in Wellington which was going to publish it. Here it was re-written by a member of the staff. In its published form (*Gentlemen of the Jury*, New Plymouth, Thomas Avery, 1937) it was a very bad book. I know of only one extant copy, and as it is in a public library my conscience has to leave it there. The theme of the book was that an illegitimate child was preferable to a dangerous abortion. The method of achieving this was to bash the abortionist. No book could survive such a *non sequitur*.

Her enthusiasm was a cause for wonder. Once, when discussing with me my practice, she said of her husband (quite correctly), 'Of course he's a very good doctor, Bill. Very good indeed. But he doesn't revel in it as I do.' She was formidable in argument or debate. In her autobiography *Backblocks Baby-Doctor* (London, Faber, 1955) she quotes some remarks I am reputed to have made. When I expostulated that I had never made them, she replied, 'Oh yes you did. It's the typical remark a man like you would make and you're just the sort of man who would forget it at once. Of course you said it.'

She later became Director of Maternal and Infant Welfare but it was not a success. She was too much an individualist ever to become a cog in an administrative machine. She soon resigned.

New Zealand owes her much. She laid the foundation stones for the present high eminence of obstetrics. There is no doubt that many persons now alive owe their existence to her though they may never have heard of her. She ranks in terms of national renown with Frances Hodgkins, Katherine Mansfield, Kate Sheppard and Ngaio Marsh. They had genius. She had clear vision and pertinacity.

She has created monuments in Dunedin and Auckland and the Auckland fame is now world wide. She had higher qualifications in Public Health, in Surgery, in Obstetrics and Gynaecology. She ran a practice in Taranaki, examined in Dunedin, interviewed possible professors in London, had a family of four, toured the country repeatedly talking to women about doctors or talking to doctors about women. When I reviewed her autobiography, both on radio and in *Landfall*, I praised her lack of affectation. She had a tale to tell and she told it, just as in life she had a task to do and she did it. Her country gave her an M.B.E. Its inadequacy tended to cheapen all decorations. Yet she will live safely in the keeping of the historians.

The war shadowed most of the colour out of the New Zealand landscape. There was an acute labour shortage followed by manpower enforcement, rationing of food and petrol, conscription, compulsory loans, curtailment of sport, and a general shortage of everything, including, at times, goodwill.

There was vast activity at Burnham on the site of the old industrial school. Trentham was no longer adequate for a national training school. Uniforms and army trucks filled the streets. Troops marched three abreast instead of four. On the country roads were jeeps, bren-gun carriers, scout cars. Many people knew all about the secret ammunition dumps and the hidden aerodromes except where they were. There were strange additions to the military vocabulary: echelon, camouflage, reconnaissance, security.

The medical world faced chaos. More and more medical men were drained into the forces. The work-load was enormously increased by the medical boarding. The first boards were held on the Sunday morning following the declaration of war. They continued almost daily for years, at first in the Drill Hall, and then in the gymnasium of Canterbury College. There was a moral compulsion to answer all calls for boarding. I have often paid several times my morning fee to colleagues who did my private work for the same period. We were the victims of the proximity of Burnham to Christchurch.

Recruits would arrive from all over the South Island bringing the viruses to which they were immune and passing them on to those who were not. Epidemics of influenza resulted and the resourceful Kiwi usually managed to be on leave when he succumbed, in the belief that the civilian doctor was more generous with convalescence. There was some relief when temporary hospitals were equipped at Addington and Burwood.

The remaining doctors often had to abandon most of the formal codes. To treat a colleague's patient was not a breach of ethics but a personal favour to a friend. The obstetricians tended to operate from a common pool ensuring that every patient had a doctor even though it was not the one with whom she had booked. The patients were always appreciative, sometimes amused.

An added burden was the moral one of trying to resist Government interference in the practice of medicine. This was a duty owed to the men overseas. Yet we were ill-equipped for the task. A weary few would attend our meetings and would struggle through the agenda. A certain motion would be stripped of its incongruities, rephrased, presented as an amendment, reformed till it could not offend anyone nor achieve anything. One night the debate was whether we would accept the offered capitation grant of seven and six. Most speakers approved and when the motion was about to be put one member at the back jumped to his feet (his constant reflex to a passing thought) and proposed an amendment that the sum be fifteen shillings. A few wits seconded it. The chairman, furious, had no option but to put it and it was passed almost unanimously. Another evening wasted by men too tired for solid debate.

The Canterbury Division issued a ruling that no man be allowed to start practice in Christchurch while Christchurch practitioners were overseas. Despite this the Government defiantly set up in practice two foreign refugees. Naturally they were ostracized but some years later when they were recognized as very worthy persons they were admitted to the membership of the B.M.A.

I remember very little of 1940 for event fell on event too rapidly to be particularized. I hardly ever saw my five children. I functioned mainly because of my wife, staunch and steadfast *in loco patris*, foreseeing every want, wish or whim. I was once called out at midnight and arrived home for breakfast having delivered five babies. I recorded the day's work (less memory lapses) in the day book and passed it gratefully to my accountants who kept assuring me I was doing all right. My bank confirmed this. Dr Irving's lawyers implored me not to repay all the mortgage as they could not get the money to England. I reminded them of the old days and forced it on them. The money struggle was now over and was (with prudence) never to return.

Often enough I have gone to sleep half way through writing a prescription, to the bewilderment of the patient who had not suspected an explanation so simple. Occasionally my wife would go to a film of her choice and insist on me as an escort. This was her thoughtfulness again for she knew as I knew that I would sleep right through.

In such a situation a doctor is caught like a fly in a web. He cannot refuse to answer a call, for a life might be at stake. He cannot call for help for all the medical services are taut. Despite the scepticism of Blackball, he does not belong to a union and fights his troubles singlehanded. He belongs to a profession which is the shortest-lived of all professions.

But 1940 was not unique. Today, all up and down the country are weary doctors, fighting fatigue, warding off sleep and preserving a great tradition.

In the end there was a foretaste of what would happen if the medical services broke down completely. More and more patients flooded the Outpatient Department of the hospital and transferred the chaos. Some had to do without a doctor and in the majority such cases recovered. One patient of mine sustained a coronary thrombosis while I was away, and in the nine hours before he died his family had been unable to get any doctor. We tried to keep the home fires burning, or if not burning at least smouldering.

This, I kept assuring myself, was as far as my patriotism could go – but I was not convinced.

9

Items of War

It was a different war. The enemy might not be more vicious but he was more viciously equipped. It was a global war with death swinging over the wide spaces of land, sea and air. New Zealand was no longer safely remote.

It was a war when communication across the Empire was all important and leading such communication was the radio. Daily, Big Ben called on all the faithful to listen. 'This is the BBC. Here is the news.' Over our radio came Chamberlain's announcement that a state of war existed between Germany and Great Britain and immediately the BBC fired its first propaganda shot. 'We will now continue our programme with light music from Snow White and the Seven Dwarfs.' Over the radio came the tragedies as well as the victories. 'The Admiralty regrets to announce the loss on the China coast of H.M.S. *Prince of Wales* and H. M. S. *Repulse*.' It was the radio that was used by those two magnificent architects of victory, Winston Churchill and Tommy Handley.

Probably all the eligible doctors of Christchurch volunteered for overseas and, as instructed, handed their names in to the secretary of the B.M.A. Here they were mulled over by a manpower committee, and by the Medical Officer of Health and by Army H.Q. in Wellington. My volunteering would be an empty gesture. My age was too great, my family too big, my practice too extensive. I talked it over with my wife. In the end we compromised. My name should go forward. In time of national peril no less would do. But almost certainly I would remain on the home front. And, shortly afterwards a letter from the Health Department to the local Medical Officer of Health stated that under no circumstances was I to be released from private practice. There was no answer to this. A good soldier goes where he is sent and a good civilian stays where he is put.

So, as a gesture, I joined the Territorials. If you are not selected for the team there is a little satisfaction in being ball boy or line umpire. I was posted to the 3rd Field Ambulance of which remarkable unit more will be said later.

On certain week-ends we trucked to some desolate area round the Waimakariri River and set up tents and marquees. At least the O/Rs did, they having the skill. I was of no use. Even the tents had changed – Indian marquees now instead of bell tents. On certain week days we paraded at the drill hall, called the roll in loud authoritative tones, marched noisily from one wall to the other and back again and then settled down to an examination of the medical panniers. This was the hour of the Medical Officers. The private who could correctly drive in the pegs for a marquee before it was unrolled could rarely put on a triangular bandage and keep the weight off the injured shoulder.

So my war effort was settled: jogging with the 3rd Fd. Ambulance, sitting for weary hours in the surgery trying to empty the waiting room, roaming the streets of Christchurch at night with a torch looking for house numbers, snatching meals and sleep and dreaming of the enormous holiday I was going to have when the boys came marching home again.

Suddenly, as is the pattern of war, this planned programme was disrupted, the disrupting agent being Sir Hugh Acland, a man with two personalities. There was his civilian personality in which he was the leading surgeon of Christchurch, a friendly co-operative colleague among his younger colleagues. I knew him mainly from assisting him at operations on my patients and I held him in high regard. The other personality was his military one. He was a veteran of three wars and now, a full colonel, was Deputy Director of Medical Services for Area 10. All the softness had now gone. He was rigidly loyal to the military tradition. The time for favours was past.

He saw me one day in a garage and came over. He was tall, erect, elegant in his uniform with its decorations and red tabs. I fully expected that because of my civilian status he would be in a civilian mood. Instead he said bluntly, 'Not doing much for your King and Country these days are you?'

I was aghast. I was so tired I could hardly stand. When I was able I set up my defences: Territorials, enlistment through the B.M.A., a letter on the Health Department files . . . . He dismissed them all with a wave of his hand. The B.M.A. was now inoperative. A letter to the M.O.H.? Surely I was not going to be deflected by a triviality of that sort?

'I decide who's indispensable here. I also decide on the type of man the army wants. If you are genuine you will enlist in the normal way.' And he strode off. I did not offer him a lift. It was the nearest I have ever come to being accused of having a yellow streak. Ten minutes later I had enlisted at the recruiting office – in the normal way. A few days later he rang me. I was prepared for his apologies. Instead he said:

'You're leaving for the army school in Trentham on Friday. Call in here for your vouchers.'

'But I can't. What about my practice?'

'Well, what about it?'

'And I haven't got a uniform.'

'Then get one.'

'How?'

'From your tailors.'

'But have they got military serge?'

'No, you get it from Burnham. And show some initiative man. You're going to be an army officer. Men will depend on you.'

Initiative, eh? He was twisting the knife in the wound. Initiative? All right, initiative then.

The guard at the Burnham camp refused to let me in, or to summon the quartermaster to the gate. So I drove round to the back of the camp and through a gap in the trees and so secured the materials. My tailors promised their best. I rang up some doctors and told them the circumstances. They sighed and said all right, they would do their best. I incorporated their names in a notice I pinned on the door.

Two hours before the boat-train left I was in uniform and had at last been positively identified by my children. I went down town on some mission and afar off I saw Sir Hugh wearily making for home. Here was a chance to hurl back at him his taunt about initiative. I confronted him and gave a smart salute. Automatically, he saluted back. He looked me up and down.

'What the hell d'you mean by appearing in public with buttons like those?'

From that moment I was back in the army, the same old army even though some of its Diggers were to become officers and the remaining Diggers were to become Kiwis.

Trentham engulfed us – a group of about twenty medical officers – but it was not my Trentham of old. I have photos of myself in the Trentham trenches, but the trenches had gone. The site of the bell tent, which would take seven only and resulted in the eighth, namely myself, waking on the path outside covered in snow was now occupied by a hut. I had two stars on my epaulettes but they carried less prestige than a single stripe on my left arm had done over twenty years before. Our chief instructor, a non-medical captain, was a gentleman and treated us as such. We contoured maps and placed our Regimental Aid Posts (R.A.Ps) out of reach of the enemy's shells and mortars. With compasses and tape-measures we found the spot where the bottle of beer was buried. We learned – to our astonishment – the structure of a modern army and the hierarchy of its control. We pored over the notes we were given and became acquainted with King's Regs, and the Manual of Military Law. 'What would you suggest in a situation like that, sir?' our captain might ask of me. Very gentlemanly. Almost on the same site a P.T. sergeant had once yelled at me, 'Keep your mouth shut, Number Four. You'll get your bloody guts sunburnt.'

For the first month back in Christchurch I was Medical Officer for C Block, Burnham. Then I was replaced by Hunter and he in turn by Roberton. The two who were not in camp did most of the practice of the one who was. During my term I wrote myself a leave pass every Wednesday afternoon and before returning to camp had given three lectures to the nurses at St Helen's, at Calvary and at the public hospital.

The year drifted by. Then came Pearl Harbour and general mobilization. I marched away with the rest. My wife, with better foresight than mine, began filling the pockets of my suits with moth balls, where they stayed for over five years.

At first all was confusion. Would the Japs attack New Zealand? If so, when and where? How could a territorial army and a suggested Home Guard dispose its defences? The map of Canterbury began to be dotted with small groups of soldiers strategically placed. I was sent to Ashburton with about a dozen men to select a site for an R.A.P. and to set it up I picked the Domain and we erected tents, removed squares of turf, dug holes, established latrines and an ablution block. No one challenged us. This was barely completed when we received orders to go back to Burnham. At Burnham we met the 3rd Fd. Ambulance, with Lieutenant-Colonel Hunter as Commanding Officer, moving down to establish a new camp at Rakaia.

A whole volume could be written on the Rakaia camp, which became the medical training school for the South Island. Here the raw drafts of civilians would march and drill, render first aid, transport wounded by truck or stretchers or fireman's lift, acquire a respect for King's Regs and the Manual of Military Law, and learn the measures to be taken with hunger, thirst and capture by the enemy.

The camp is here presented only as an *aide-mémoire* to those who were there. The majority will remember the Maori House, our only recreation edifice, ninety-six feet long, made of bluegum posts, rusty wire from the river bed, sheaves of broom for walls and roof, and windows made of X-ray plates, by courtesy of Calvary Hospital. Fewer will know of its finances. The total cost was two and ninepence (mainly nails) made up of two and six found in the Y.M.C.A. and a donation of threepence from some officer who hoped to be named as a patron.

Few participants will have forgotten the six weeks at the upper Rakaia gorge practising water transport on our own patent of four stretchers and a tarpaulin (a method later used with success at Casino, so I have been informed). They will remember the winter storms that flattened all our tents till tent pegs had to be replaced by transverse logs in trenches below the level of the liquid mud. And the blocked silage pit by the kitchen which finally failed to respond to Captain McCombs' dynamite, necessitating a drain towards the river. The levels were secured by a homemade theodolite devised by the transport officer, Bob Smith, his basic component being a .303 rifle. They would not forget how we rescued the pedigree sheep marooned in the swirl of a Rakaia flood. Or how when the floods ripped up the railway approaches to the bridge the north and south bound traffic continued, the gap being filled by the trucks of 3rd Fd. Amb. Or our share in the harvesting of mid-Canterbury where if a farmer applied for two stookers for a fortnight he would be sent fifty men for half a day; or our R.A.Ps so well camouflaged in the gorse of the Rakaia river bed that I, flying with the pilot, could not identify them; or the course in weapon-training, rifles, machine guns, anti-tank rifles and hand-grenades for all ranks, with revolver practice for the officers.

Rakaia was a special type of camp with an unusual autonomy. The C.O. and his staff made up the weekly training syllabus. Copies sent to Sir Hugh and the D.A.D.M.S., Colonel Woodhouse, were received without comment. The camp had few buildings or facilities. As a result the officers lived close to the men. Hunter and I had pledged ourselves that we would never ask the men to do anything that we would not attempt ourselves. There were times when the heroism of this outshone the wisdom. Once, during elaborate manoeuvres on the barren mid-Canterbury plains, I marched with A Company for twenty-five miles on each of three consecutive days. At the end I dared not stop for the hourly break for fear the engine would not start again. But eventually my elephantine plodding on flat feet brought me to the camp gates.

The camp was well served by its officers. The quartermaster was Captain McCombs (now Sir Terence McCombs). He was probably the most capable quartermaster in the country and was the originator of a number of new techniques. As a Member of Parliament his influence was wide. The Adjutant was the ebullient Arthur ('Shorty') Martin, later Assistant Registrar of Canterbury College. The rare distinction of being a non-medical officer in a medical unit fell to Captain A. Crowther, Professor of Psychology at Canterbury College. Lieutenant R. Smith of the Christchurch Tramway staff was our transport officer and he transformed the mechanics of locomotion into an art. A key position in the day-to-day routine of the camp was that of Senior Dispenser, held by Sergeant Sherlock, now of Iggos, chemists of Cashel Street. We also had Private Clifton Cook, the despair of sergeants and the delight of musicians.

When Colonel Hunter went overseas as commanding officer of the 7th Fd. Amb. and Major Roberton had returned to civil practice I became C.O. of the 3rd Fd. Amb. I maintained a serious training programme finding a positive satisfaction in organization. Because of my previous experience in the ranks I could the more easily understand the O/Rs. There has to be distinction between officers and men but the distinction should be a military one only as denoted by rank. In the army, efficiency has to be assured by a few being dressed in a little brief authority.

Men came and went and eventually the camp numbers fell, particularly to the 10th Reinforcements, where officers and men voluntarily surrendered rank so as to be included in the draft. 'We have kept all our reinforcements up,' said General Bowerbank from Wellington. 'But I don't know where we get the men from.' Colonel Acland knew. 'Don't you tell him,' he ordered me.

As our field activities shrank our administration increased. Every week we had to supply about thirty-five returns, hardly any of them with relevance to us or our camp. I wrote in expostulation to Colonel Woodhouse, an intemperate letter which I regretted as soon as it was past recall. Benign and polite, he wrote back trying to justify his returns, but he was wrong on his facts and even more wrong on his deductions. This angered me and fuel to the anger was that he had just asked for a return of returns. I failed to see that his temperate letter was also a lesson in good manners. So I wrote back, recklessly, even belligerently. Hasty judgements are always wrong, as I realized the next day. This time there would have to be a repercussion.

A week later the throaty voice of Colonel Acland came over the phone.

'Is that you, Bennett? Are you prepared to drop rank and go overseas at short notice?'

'Yes, sir.'

'That's just as well. Because you're going whether you like it or not.'

Rakaia closed. The few personnel and their assets returned to Burnham. The vehicles went to Addington, there being just enough drivers in camp with heavy truck licences. This included me. The Rakaia folk moved back into their Domain and burned down the Maori House and swept our traces away. Ichabod, Ichabod.

The 3rd Fd. Amb. has never had a reunion. It never had enough permanency. It was like a Casualty Clearing Station. The men came in, suffering from being civilians, and were cured of that, equipped with some knowledge and passed on. Over thirty years later it is still remembered. Patients, war pensioners, casual acquaintances. . . 'I was with you in Rakaia'. I think, by most, it is kindly remembered.

The Liberty ship that took us to Nouméa presumably interpreted its liberty as the right to toss and roll in a faultless sea. On board were masses of Americans and a few New Zealanders, about thirty of whom were returning after leave. They had been this way before and I had not, yet I, being a captain, commanded them. It was an easy responsibility. Both at Wellington and at Auckland I had given them all-night leave in return for a word-of-honour promise from each man that he would be on the station at the named hour the next morning. There were no defaulters.

The beautiful harbour of Nouméa contracted down to the little crowded cosmopolitan wharf. Like all tropical scenes it was full of colour. Prominent in the crush and confusion on the wharf were New Zealand trucks driven by nonchalant independent New Zealanders. The Kiwi rank and file rapidly adapts to new surroundings be it desert or jungle or anything in between. Our driver was a slap-happy private keen to get going. Our destination was N.Z. Headquarters at Bourail nearly two hundred miles away. We sat on long wooden boards fixed to either side of the truck. Soon we were all standing. Boards that fling you in the air and then rise to meet your descent can be disconcerting. Our driver hugged the right hand side of the road, scorned corners, ignored potholes and seemed to believe that the essence of good driving was speed.

Bourail, a picturesque small French village with a few white-washed houses on either side of the road was reached after midnight, and the day concluded with a meal and the disposal of aching limbs on camp stretchers. The next morning I had a long interview with the D.D.M.S., Colonel J. M. Twhigg of Wellington, and learned for the first time the military situation in New Caledonia (abbreviated to Necal). I had been posted to the 22nd Fd. Amb. as Second in Command (2 I/C). Later in the day I travelled the twenty-odd miles to the camp, which was in a bush clearing and near a stream. The unit was mainly a North Island one and few of the personnel were known to me with the exception of the C.O. Lieutenant-Colonel W. F. Shirer, also of Wellington. We had been students together. The Adjutant was the very active L. H. Hudson and the genial Quartermaster J. Betteridge. Medical Officers included Captain Ferguson, Captain Simpson, Captain Clouston, Captain Tuckey, Lieutenant Lang. Attached to the Field Ambulance was the No. 1 Field Surgical Unit commanded by Major P. Brunette with Captain Ryder as his assistant. Also attached was a wing of the Army Service Corps.

It was a unit quite different from the 3rd Fd. Amb. where the personnel came and went and reserved their loyalty for something more stable. The 22nd was closely knit. It had seen service in Fiji and had had long tough training in New Zealand.

I arrived to a camp completely disorganized as the final preparations were being made for the shift to the forward area. I could contribute little to this and was sent back to Nouméa to organize some stores. I travelled at night in a jeep. My elderly driver took sick after a few miles and I left him at another small New Zealand unit on the way. It was easier controlling the jeep than controlling the road. Repeatedly at corners I would confront an American convoy and shoot over urgently to the right and drive through a blast of American profanity.

Nouméa at close quarters was not attractive. Its most impressive buildings were enormous American storehouses. The Americans dominated Necal. They also dominated the Third New Zealand Expeditionary Force supplying us with equipment, food, weapons, transport and a variety of military orders. We were bound for Guadalcanal, but all our transport lingered for a week at Vila in the New Hebrides, where we underwent intensive amphibious training.

Any American training is rigorous. At midnight the siren would call. To dress would take about thirty seconds, then laden with gear we would scramble down the rope nets into the boats and race for the shore. The late-comer, the man in difficulties, the one who slipped on the ropes, was left to extricate himself as best he could. On the shore we had to splash through the surf, assemble in the jungle, and then execute some operation order in the dark. Here for the first time we met one of our two enemies, malarial mosquitoes.

We reached Guadalcanal and on a limited camp site the unit reassembled. A main military road ran through the camp. It was all very beautiful with the sea on one side, jagged cliffs on the other, scattered patches of exotic trees and jungles, all gay with the colours of the tropics.

But there was no human contribution to the beauty. That first night we watched a lone Jap bomber, a little black beetle in the blaze of searchlights, chugging to Henderson airfield where it dropped its bombs and then returned. There were no night-fighters and apparently no anti-aircraft fire. Yet the land was ours. Our camp was on part of one of the great battlegrounds of history where the southern sweep of the Japs had been stopped and a base formed for the slow beat back to Tokyo. All over the area were dumps of shells and machine gun belts. Just above high water mark was a series of dugouts. Conspicuously placed on many a parapet was a hand-grenade so obviously inviting investigation that the investigation was denied till the engineers had proved they were not booby traps.

All over the area was mute evidence of a beaten Japanese army doggedly trying to avert its final destruction. From high up on the hills down to the beach were their dumps of discarded equipment. First they piled their gasmasks, then their heavier shells, next their machine gun ammunition and finally their grenades and items of personal equipment. The stamp of the victors was also there. Piles of heavier shells, discarded American ammunition cases and fully charged machine gun belts. (Quite a few of these had been buried, inviting much speculation as to the reason.)

It was no Pyrrhic victory. Offshore at an angle on the coral were the tips of many wrecked Japanese landing craft. Further out, every few days a convoy of freighters would arrive from America and the amphibious trucks ('ducks') would swim out alongside, receive their loads and return to shore. All night the noise and clamour persisted. By morning the seas were clear; the convoy had gone; the road through our camp rattled and shook day and night with heavy American trucks. The road was later widened at our expense from two lanes to four lanes. Before this happened I (then Acting C.O. as Colonel Shirer was away on a reconnaissance) decided to protest against not being allowed to retain our camp of approximately half a square mile among the two thousand five hundred square miles of Guadalcanal. My search for the Island Command was vain. The best I could do was an appointment for the next day. When I returned to camp the road was already through and on its edge was my tent, brown with dust. At the entrance was a Jap skeleton, spreadeagled intact by the last bulldozer and soon to be buried by the next.

That the camp was strewn with ammunition of all types and occupied by non-combatant troops gave rise to some anxiety. All medical units should have weapon training as the 3rd Fd. Amb. had in Rakaia. Such training is not to facilitate their use of weapons but to prevent their abuse. All military records have their stories where ignorance of weapons has caused military disasters. Yet the 22nd Fd. Amb. had been together a long time and to them the discipline of arms was part of their general knowledge. The officers, when outside the camp precincts, had to carry revolvers.

I know of only one instance in this camp where caution failed. Two privates, clambering up a wooded hill at the back of the camp came on an artillery dump. On the top was a large shell which appeared bright and new. One man picked it up. His mate advised caution. 'Throw it away,' he said. Which, incredibly, the other did, literally, nose-cap down. The resultant explosion seemed to shake the whole island. But the shell had been thrown behind the trunk of a large tree. The tree was shattered but it provided a thin arc of safety in which the two men were standing. No one was injured. There was talk of bringing an orderly room charge against them so that they would not do it again. I intervened. I had seen them, shocked, shaking and speechless. I guaranteed that they would not do it again.

The Japs did not respect the medical services, nor the Red Cross, and had not been a signatory to the appropriate Geneva Convention. On the road two hundred yards beyond our camp they had ambushed a party of unarmed American stretcher bearers and had slaughtered them and their patients while the Americans watched helplessly from the hill tops. How different it might have been had the stretcher bearers been armed or had an armed escort. It was over this spot that the Americans erected a huge banner across the road, 'Kill the bastards'. Later in the forward areas of Green Island and Nissan the O/Rs of both the 7th and 22nd Fd. Ambulances were issued with rifles and grenades, which were willingly accepted even by some pacifists.

Guadalcanal was only a transit camp. We acted as headquarters for the medical services of the 14th Brigade, kept a tidy camp under difficult conditions and, when possible, trained for the arduous days ahead. This involved on one occasion an all day route march for A Company with myself as the Company Commander accompanying them. This was a reckless decision on account of my age, my unfit state and the weight I had to carry. I had my haversack, water bottle, binoculars, compass, map case, revolver and six rounds. This was all light enough for the first hour till the slopes got steeper, the spear-like grass was taller, the coral surface dangerously uneven. My sergeant sensed my limitations. (How little can an officer hide from an intelligent sergeant.) By mutual yet unvoiced agreement the control of the march passed from me to him. Yet, by forfeiting the hourly break I was more or less with them when the midday halt was made. It was a pleasant level area, heavily wooded at the mouth of a valley down which a river ran. On one side of the valley was a nearly vertical cliff face. This worried me. There was as yet no proof that the area was free of Japs and the top of the cliff would be a perfect ambush setting. Nearby was a group of noisy Americans, but there was nothing reassuring about them. In order to investigate, I decided to climb a nearby tree higher than the cliff itself. This I did and satisfied myself that beyond the cliff were only spare stunted trees and no cover for Japs. I began to descend when there came a burst of machine fire and a few feet below me branches of the tree were slashed. I swung to the other side. If this was hostile fire it was coming from the wrong angle. I slipped down a few branches but was halted by another burst just below me. I made two more essays and there were two more bursts. Then I saw him. He was an American sitting with his back to a tree, a submachine gun in his hands and a grin on his face. I let him see that he was discovered and he let me descend unmolested.

I strode over, and blew my wrath on him. He continued to be amused and showed no contrition. I realized that to him I was only another of these curious half-civilized New Zealanders. We wore no badges of rank in the field. He summed the whole incident up: 'Gee, you was a scared guy, you was'. And he was a correct guy, he was.

The transfer to Vella Lavella was a smooth procedure. The Americans wrote the operation order and I, as Acting C.O., passed it on to the junior officers and sergeants and all was well. We travelled in a convoy of twenty-two destroyers. I can describe only mine. It was an animated collection of metals, hot, cramped, noisy and heavily armed. Most of our troops slept on the bare deck and during the first night were rewarded with a fireworks display in New Georgia where a heavy Jap raid was concentrated on Munda airfield. By day the decks were unbearably hot and it was necessary to keep moving even in rubber-soled shoes. The Americans decided that it was a suitable day to hold a full-scale gunnery practice. (Surely no noise is more devastating than naval guns a few feet away.)

The other diversion of that day was that it was election day in New Zealand. A tarpaulin was stretched across two gun turrets to make a booth. One by one we appeared before the Returning Officer, Lieutenant Hudson, assisted by three poll clerks, sergeants from A Company. In turn we declared our home electorate, were shown the list of candidates and so voted. The Americans were amazed – no speeches, no streamers, no camouflage, no expenses. The Japs might have been perturbed. The enemy, far from being cowed, was going into battle flaunting his loyalty to the democracy of the Homeland.

The Americans were further amazed because we voted on the liquor question. American naval ships are dry and the thirsty have a choice of coffee or chlorinated water. Despite the heat and the sweat one man declared that he intended to vote for prohibition. A sergeant, outraged took him behind a gun turret and finally converted him to right thinking. The sergeant then recorded his own vote so casually and confidently that he crossed out the wrong line.

In the morning we came to Vella Lavella, a low-lying purple arc on the horizon, indistinguishable from any other of the thousands of islands in the Pacific. We had air-cover but, surprisingly, there was no resistance, on sea, air or land. The ships anchored outside the reef. We scrambled down into the LSTs (landing ships, tanks) which then rushed to the shore. Immediately the destroyers departed. We splashed through the surf onto the beach, a narrow coral strip flanked at either end by trees growing even in the salt water of the high tides. Behind the strand of beach was the jungle, dense, dripping, teeming, mysterious and awesome.

Each unit had managed to land at least one truck. We followed the drill and reassembled as a unit. Colonel Shirer was waiting and led us through the jungle and its cloying slush to our camp site in Gill's Plantation two miles away.

The rest of that day saw the Ambulance at its best. It trampled down the head-high undergrowth, raised the tents, hacked mess-tables out of the jungle, erected a hospital, set out the signs and changed confusion into a fully functioning unit. Our truck held cooking gear. That night, we dined unsuspectingly on spam and dehydrated potatoes. Within two hours of our arrival a man with an acute appendix was sent in from another unit. The surgical unit was still erecting tents, but paused long enough to remove the appendix.

The next morning the enemy arrived, air-borne, and were challenged by R.N.Z.A.F. fighter squadrons. Spasmodically throughout the day the battles raged, now out at sea, now over our heads. Sometimes as many as a dozen planes would be weaving and diving, making split-second decisions. The enemy were trying to attack a second convoy bringing heavier equipment, but could not pierce the air defence. At least seven Jap planes were shot down (official figures). The battles were breathlessly followed by the men of the 14th Brigade, all closely congregated in their units. It was a grand curtain raiser. What our chaps could do in the air we could do on land. For the next few days there were desultory dogfights. Thereafter our only threats were from the bombers.

A week or two of camp life, defects and deficiencies slowly being corrected, roads and paths constructed, more undergrowth cleared, camp chores, sick parade, routine orders, spam and dehydrated potatoes. It was a time full of incident but lacking in drama. To me, Vella Lavella was one of the ecological mysteries of the Pacific. In a narrow section of the vast past it must have been a coral excrescence above a level sea. Then came. . . what? Seaweed and marine dross and tide-borne seeds. A primitive vegetation must have resulted and on this was founded the present mat of choking vegetation fighting parasitically for sun and air and survival. It grows from its own compost, several feet deep, brownish black, rotting rank-smelling. How could this nutrient soil increase at a greater rate than the growth that supplied it? And how could it differentiate into its species, mahogany (which we used for bridges) and soft-growing kauri?

The jungle vibrates with life. Force your way into it and snakes rustle off. Land crabs almost as large as dinner plates move tortuously over the debris. Everywhere is the insect life, and leading it all, in numbers, aggressiveness and omniscience is the little black ant. It truly lives to eat. It is said that there are over four and a half thousand species of ant, of which one must be peculiar to the Solomons. No food is safe except in the closest fitting tins. The legs of our mess tables were set in tins of water but before long ants were walking over a bridge of dead ants and the sugar tin on the table was black. Long columns will wind up a coconut tree and having gorged on nectar will descend, being now twice the size. On the basis of the relative sizes of a man and an ant this is equivalent to a man instinctively sensing food nearly seven miles away. I once caught and chloroformed a magnificent butterfly and was determined to get it back to New Zealand. I pinned it out on a piece of cardboard which dangled by two linen threads to another thread bridging the clear space between two trees. In the morning the mountings were untouched. The butterfly was an empty carcase. Among the ants are often to be found black beetles, majestically secure in weight and carapace. But, as I have seen several times, if a beetle moves feebly, or tilts to one side, ants come racing from all directions. They pile on the moving growing mound. Round the periphery is a chaos of ants arriving and ants departing. At length the heap breaks up and the area clears, leaving no trace of any beetle.

All life must have begun in the Pacific, despite the biologists. It has a tempo designed for nascent things. Nothing is static. The clouds race, the deluge falls, the giants of the jungle crash, the sky clears, the hermit crabs come out of the tides to cover the beach. High up, the parakeets fly and often iguanas move. Below are the snakes and rats and crabs. In mid-air are the butterflies and the mosquitoes. And always in the wet spongy soil is the thrust of new life.

Some of our men said they could see the young coconut palms growing. It was an exaggeration but not as gross as many soldiers' tales. Some letters from New Zealand carried a few small seeds, of flowers and vegetables. Outside the tents they grew magnificently, almost incredibly. And in a few weeks when harvest was near they would droop and in a day would be rotting back into the warmth again.

We took our showers in the almost daily deluge. It was a simple matter of kicking off our footwear, shedding two garments and stepping out of the tent with a cake of soap. Towelling was perfunctory. Skin and clothes were perpetually moist.

The Japs on the island were estimated at one thousand. Opposing them was the 35th Battalion which began hopping from bay to bay, securing minor beachheads and pressing the enemy back. The details of the campaign need not feature here. Two or three hundred Japs were killed. The rest escaped in small boats. Garrison duties followed at strategic points round the island. Close behind the battalion during the fighting the Field Ambulance supplied an R.A.P. With this went Colonel Shirer and Lieutenant Hudson. I was left in camp which was against my wishes and against standard practice. Of our men, thirty-two were killed in action and thirty-one wounded. In addition there were many American casualties and a grim incidence of tropical ills. The wounded who came to us from the jungle had simple bullet wounds. Much different were the bomb casualties. On one occasion some New Zealanders and Americans were unloading ships on the beach. Two Japanese dive-bombers evaded the cover and dropped their bombs on the deck. The casualties, dreadful cases of amputated limbs, gaping flaps of flesh, brutal baring of anatomy and the choking, sucking wounds of the chest, came to us from a mile away, the trucks grinding up the coral road.

We had what we called bomb-proof wards – excavated areas three feet deep to take as many stretchers as a marquee would cover. It was effective against bomb fragments but not against a direct hit. Here the recoverable cases went, soon overflowing into neighbouring tents. Two tents were erected for the dead. The Field Surgical Unit was operating continuously. For much of the time I was their anaesthetist, relying on intravenous avertin as the volatile anaesthetics were unsuitable in that heat. The efficiency of the Ambulance was admirable. Hardly any orders were given. Every man had his job, usually self-selected, and he moved quickly, quietly and confidently. It was a situation often reviewed in training and was faithfully enacted in the actual crisis.

Sickness was rife. Dermatitis – the product of heat, sweat and salt – affected thousands of men. Bacillary dysentery was in epidemic form, and some of the fighting squads so badly affected that, had the Japs known, the results could have been serious. We used enormous quantities of sulphaguanadine. There was a steady trickle of malaria, despite the malarial drill. I was sent on a tour of the island with a supply officer and on one headland there was a garrison force of eleven, nine of whom had infective hepatitis.

We were poorly fed. Everything came from American tins, and naturally did not include any delicacies, though on Thanksgiving Day we were supplied with more turkey than we could eat. The standby was spam, with tins of M. & B. (meat and beans) and M. & V. (meat and vegetables). The meat was merely an advertising gimmick. On two occasions at least the men paraded with their tin plates and there was no food. A supply ship had tangled with a bomber. In one bay I saw thousands of tins, all labels gone, bobbing against the coral cliffs. There was no fruit on the island. The charm of coconut milk went on the third day. Parcels from home were regular and precious. There was also fish. One hand grenade thrown from the reef once resulted in over four hundred fish. Fishing by this method was strictly forbidden, said the officers who ate heartily of the fish. I once came down the coast in a storm-tossed LST along with some Americans, some New Zealanders and one miserable dejected Jap prisoner. Someone suggested he might be hungry and he was given an open tin of M. & B. He was ravenous, scooping it out of the tin with his fingers. A little later he was violently sick. 'You see,' we said to the Americans. 'As we told you. Even a Jap . . . .'

The tour round the island was a protracted one, for we were wrecked on a reef and were the guests of an American Radar Unit for a week. When I arrived back at camp I found that Colonel Shirer had been recalled to New Zealand for civilian duties. He was a popular officer and his going was regretted. His efficiency was recognized by his being mentioned in despatches. The 22nd Fd. Ambulance had a total of four commanding officers; at the regular reunions since, Colonel Shirer automatically presides.

I became the new C.O. Were any radical changes necessary? I knew of none. But I did know of the danger to morale when front line troops know nothing of their future. Look after the morale and the efficiency looks after itself.

So I went morale-building. Natives were engaged to build a recreational *bure* (wages stipulated by Headquarters to be a shilling a day). Each day two men were allowed twenty-four hours leave. There was nothing for them to do and nowhere to go but it showed good intentions. The first two decided to visit the American Air Field. That evening the Air Field rang up to say there had been some heavy bombing and two bodies were unidentified. Had we lost two bodies? For a dreadful few minutes we had, and then they walked in, having left a few minutes before the bombing.

I started a magazine, *The Larynx*. It was typed on the orderly room typewriter, the pages stapled together and pinned to a coconut tree. Here it was available for anyone sufficiently interested. I wrote one article on our cooks who worked in appalling conditions in the mud. I prophesied that, the war over, they would return to Vella Lavella to guide tourists. The cooks were not amused, and when they were taunted by some of the men on a mess parade, a free fight developed with spam and mush of potatoes flying through the air.

A rifle contest was arranged, and surprisingly almost every man in the unit wanted to compete. I, unable to wear glasses in that humidity, could not see the targets. As a result I achieved probably the worst score of all and there is no doubt that this decidedly improved the morale.

Occupational therapy was encouraged. The Kiwi is a genius at improvisation. First he had to get a hacksaw, a file, an auger and a couple of sheets of sandpaper. In this he was invariably successful. ('The Americans can always get more.') Then he surrounded himself with fancy timber, brass, tortoiseshell, monumental ivory nut, leather, Japanese parachutes, and turned out ornate daggers, jewel cases and model ships. My request for recreational tools was refused.

My satisfaction in commanding a unit in the forward area never quite fulfilled its high promise. General Barrowclough informed us that he had no idea of the future of the 14th Brigade. We were living ascetically with hardly any amenities. That we should be permanently on garrison duties behind the Americans was a melancholy thought. In such circumstances the morale rapidly deteriorates. Later I was in a position to review the neurosis and psychosis of the 3rd Division. A constant incidence of these in time of inactivity was followed by a decrease when the troops learned they were going into action.

I also had to admit to less military fervour than I had in the first war. To me, one of the most disturbing procedures of war is to see troops lined up on foreign shores waiting for embarkation. Drab, exclusively masculine, trained killers going out over the horizon with the sole purpose of spoiling and killing. In any rational philosophy of mankind, where do they fit in? And what are the consequences? Round us was all the tawdry discarded equipment of war. Out on the reef were a dozen or so wrecked vessels. I was summoned one night to the next door camp where a relief guard going on duty did not hear the challenge and had most of his heart shot away. Near our camp an American plane had nose-dived into the liquid mud of the jungle and was now buried in it at an unknown depth. Was the pilot down there too? Certainly the pilot was down there, pinpointed by the many rat holes on the surface. Off-shore I saw bloated Jap corpses just below the surface slowly turning over and over in the current. And in the fulness of time all the surviving combatants go home with flags waving and crowds cheering, which is right and proper because they have been brave men. My melancholy in no way affected my loyalty. I would fight the Japs as zealously as I would fight the streptococcus but I could deplore the necessity to fight either.

Then suddenly I lost my command. A reconnaissance party from Headquarters, in which I was included, went to the small island of Baga about twenty miles away to verify that the Japs had forsaken it. They

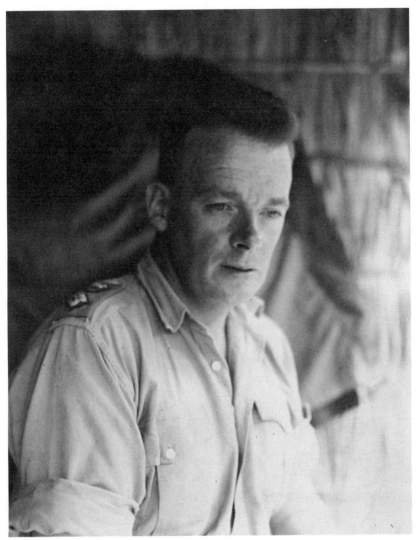

Lietenant-Colonel Bennett, Pacific, 1944

apparently had, and halfway round the circuit of the island I asked permission of the Brigadier to return over the top of the island. He agreed. There ensued a lamentable two hours packed with such misfortunes as falling down a cliff; detouring crazily to avoid other cliffs; a wildly swinging compass; getting lost; doing the appropriate drill when one is lost and still remaining lost; being unable to see anything through the jungle except the sun, which seemed to be on the wrong side of the island;

finding a deep trail through long grass on a plateau, as if a body had been dragged, and changing this theory when in jumping across a sluggish stream further on I nearly put my foot on a crocodile. The only thing that functioned was my watch, inexorably swinging round to the rendezvous time at the boat. When it arrived and I seemed to be imprisoned in impenetrable jungle I fired my revolver. A distant faint 'Coo-ee' answered. It was from a most improbable quarter yet I made for it. The call came again and I replied. The distance narrowed. The calling went on. At length I stumbled down a ravine and found the sea, the shore and a Brigade officer. 'Sorry, old man but I'm afraid you're for it. The Brig.'s fuming. Can you run?'

I couldn't run but I did. It was nearly half a mile to the LST. The prow snapped up behind me and we were off. I gasped some apologies to the Brigadier and then stretched out on my back fighting for breath as I had once done in Ewshott camp and on a messroom form in the *Athenic*. There was no chance of dissembling my distress from the rest. We reached Vella Lavella. I had sufficiently recovered to be able to apologize again to the Brigadier and to climb into a jeep.

I knew my position was in danger. But none of them were medical men. To them I could have been a valiant soldier fighting his way through the jungle to a stage of exhaustion. As long as the D.D.M.S. did not know . . . . And the next morning John Twhigg said, 'Well, how's the asthma?' Two days later he advised, 'I'm getting Barrowclough to take your place. We want you as a physician in the General Hospital in Necal.'

I could not protest. The forward area is for the fit only. There is enough morbidity there without importing it. A man not fit lacks efficiency, is liable to be a burden and may be a menace if he encounters the enemy's intelligence service. My company made me a present of a decorated Japanese shell which was touching, though illegal.

The 4th General Hospital in the Dumbéa Valley, within easy reach of Nouméa was the base hospital for 3 Division. It was well-equipped with prefabricated wards, operating theatre and departments for radiology, bacteriology, pathology and pharmacy. The O.C. was Colonel Sayers (now Sir Edward Sayers).

But most of the New Zealand troops were in the northern half of the island, two or three hundred miles away over difficult roads. So a subsidiary hospital had been established at a place called Kalavere, a few miles north of Bourail. The site was already laid out, being an old American base. There were four large wards of light wooden construction as well as the other offices of a hospital. Roads, paths, cookhouse, mess *bures* and administration buildings were taken over. The patients were derived from neighbouring units, passing Americans and the native French population, male and female. A surgeon and nursing staff were supplied from the 4th General. Also, in the same grounds, was No. 1 Convalescent Depot, devoted to rehabilitation. The O.C. of both the hospital and the convalescent unit was Lieutenant-Colonel Wood. He had arrived with his personnel from New Zealand in time to complete the second half of the hospital structure. When hospital and depot were smoothly functioning, Lieutenant-Colonel Wood incurred some severe pulmonary infection, and after a short illness, he died. This was on the day I left Guadalcanal for Necal. John Twhigg arrived from Vella Lavella the following day and two days later informed me that I was now O.C. of Kalavere hospital and attached Convalescent Depot and that I was to leave by jeep in an hour.

I arrived late in the afternoon. My driver shouted at the guards on the gate and they reluctantly let us through. I went into the orderly room. There was no one there. I strolled through the camp. There were many troops about and some gazed curiously. I wore more or less the clumsy apparel of Vella Lavella, my kitbag being still in the store in Bourail.

It was a pleasant place, once the site of the 109th American General Hospital. The ground was undulating and there was no undergrowth, no litter, no eyesores. A well kept, tidy camp. The site was fringed with trees and in them were clusters of tents. Up the hill, geographically isolated, were the tents for the Sisters and members of the Voluntary Aid Detachment (VADs). Scattered along the paths were boxes of oranges and bananas. Secretly I pocketed two oranges. Oh, for the chance of scattering oranges among the boys on Vella. I went back to the orderly room. A tall, fairheaded lieutenant named Hugh Williams admitted to being the Quartermaster. In turn, I confessed to being the new O.C. He seemed surprised but did not dispute it. My second tour round the camp was in a jeep, meeting, inspecting, asking and listening. Of the officers, the chief medical man was Captain Sealey Wood (now surgeon of Auckland), a most conscientious doctor and one of high social value because of his temperament and his skill with the violin. As I was to discover later an important asset to the unit was the lively and energetic Army Education Welfare officer, Ted Spragon. The Adjutant was Captain Mackie. We also had Padre Froude, and Lieutenants Hobson and Cato. The Matron was Miss Gunn. All the Sisters and officers dined together in a wide-open *bure*. I went to bed early that night in my own *bure* where an American General had once slept. I ate four oranges. I was apparently the only one left in camp with any taste for such fruit. I went to sleep quietly satisfied. I had already recognized in some of the personnel the enthusiasm that determines a good unit. It was shut away from the blast of war, secure and uneventful.

Before midnight the Adjutant woke me. One of the VADs had been killed in a truck accident. These same orderlies again illustrated the adaptability of the Kiwi abroad. Many of them made rapid progress in learning French and were welcome visitors at French farmhouses. In contrast to the quiet hospital the convalescent depot hummed with activity. The days were fragmented into strict schedules, of drill, ball games, gymnastics, but there were many other aspects, cultural, educational, diversionary. The N.C.O.s responsible were picked men, full of enthusiasm and imagination. The equipment, specially in the Con. Depot, was on a generous scale. It included a number of bicycles which were monopolized by the Fijians. They swept dangerously down the hill, puffed their way up again, and accompanied it all with laughter and shouting. The amusement of Fijians is refreshingly simple and pure. One day I questioned one of them as to why his countrymen were fascinated with bicycles. He was an intelligent man and gave the matter deep thought, and finally gave his opinion: 'I think Fijians just like riding bikes'.

We were under the control of the Officer in Charge of Administration (O.I.C.A.), Brigadier Dove. He was a martinet inclined at times to confuse efficiency (which was his end) with discipline (which was his means). But no dictatorship has ever sat comfortably on the Kiwi in the mass.

A new broom sweeps clean, but if there is nothing to sweep the broom still hangs. I made a few changes in detail but mainly kept a benign supervision of the *status quo*. There was a vast deal of administrative work and most of my day was spent in the orderly room.

Meanwhile in the forward area the 14th Brigade had occupied Green Island and the 8th Brigade had taken Nissan in the Treasuries. Thereafter the Americans stated that they could see no further combative role for the 3rd Division. The men began to come back to Necal, landing north of Kalavere. They brought the sick with them and we became busier.

Kalavere in this chronicle exists now in isolated memories. There was a Kiwi Concert party. ('Mares eat oats and does eat oats', 'Now is the Hour', 'Coming In on a Wing and a Prayer'), a race meeting with French horses and New Zealand jockeys and gullible Americans, where three days before I had seen, but had not believed, the complete list of the winners; a wedding, where one of our Sisters married a combatant officer, and O.I.C.A. made a gracious speech and presentation, and I gave the bride away and posed with Matron Gunn as the distressed parents, 'facing the twilight of our years together'.

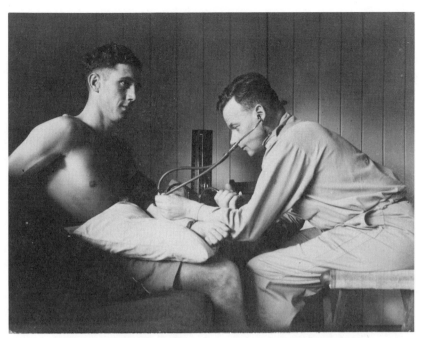

Lt-Col Bennett examining a patient, Kalavere Hospital, 1944

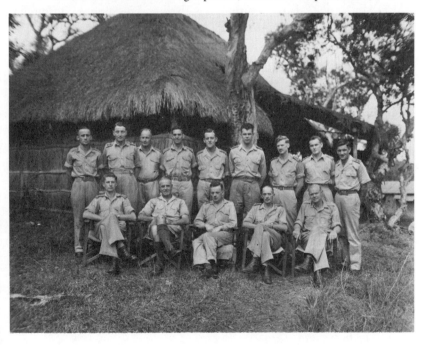

Kalavere Hospital, 1944; Lt-Col Bennett seated, centre front

One Sunday morning all unit commanders were summoned to a conference at Headquarters. The Third Division, so the O.I.C.A. informed us, was to be broken up. Some would stay on garrison duties, some would go to the Middle East. The majority would go back to New Zealand to work in agricultural pursuits. Food was becoming more important than fighters. No man would be forced against his will. And it was all top secret. No hint was to be given even to 2 I/Cs until 1800 hours that evening, when all O.C.s would address their troops. I went back and called the meeting. No one in the camp learned anything of its purpose from me. Yet, that evening when the bell rang and some hundreds started trooping into the *bure*, they set up a chorus of farming noises, an artistic blending of the animal range from the high whinny of a stallion down to the wail of a tomcat. It indicated some gross breach of security. It also indicated that it is not easy to hoodwink the Kiwi.

So they began to drift away. The hospital was half empty. The Con. Depot lost interest in fighting for fitness when there was no fighting to do. They were grey days. I had been at the death of the 3rd Fd. Amb., at the stagnation of 22nd Fd. Amb. and now apparently was to preside over the demise of Kalavere Hospital.

Suddenly, when that demise still seemed far away, I received orders to proceed to New Zealand on furlough with three days' notice. Furlough is precious. Leave is only a privilege but furlough implies a reward for service. It also implied that I would be coming back. I had not volunteered to return to New Zealand in any agricultural capacity. I had milked my last cow long before.

My wife met me at Auckland, having discovered the time and place by a method I know not, though I suspect Sir Hugh Acland. At home the family had grown predictably in height and personality. To them I, *in absentia*, had acquired some prestige. Now with some of my old characteristics surfacing, they had to change the image but, loyally, they did so slowly. A man goes to war, say the orators, for the sake of King and Country. But most go to war for the sake of their wives and kids, which is the same thing in nearer focus.

My wife reminded me of the spade I had bought her before I left. She then led me to the rear of the house. The old croquet lawn had gone for ever and was replaced by a glorious green patchwork of vegetables, crisp radishes, salads galore, lusty tomato plants and confident fresh potatoes. I wished I could have added to them a few of the truckloads of oranges and bananas which the French farmers had tipped over the cliffs after I had refused to buy them.

After a week, Army Headquarters wrote. Instead of the return to Necal

I was posted to Papakura Camp as Senior Medical Officer. I could not understand this. It was neither furlough nor promotion. Was I being steadily demoted? Or was I being ordered to mark time?

It was an impressive camp: white buildings, formal streets, signposts, flags, guards, all disposed on a beautiful lawn. Every day the rain hosed down the white paint, put a little more reflection on the black asphalt paths and gave a further rinse of green to the grass. It had been drained by war. At times, small bodies of troops could be seen in the distance, weather permitting. But all the orderly rooms were busy. The ranks had gone but the files remained. My title of S.M.O. meant in effect sole medical officer. Sometimes I had help – as when the camp once suddenly flooded with troops and then in a few days emptied as another reinforcement left for the Middle East. I took sick parades, did a little boarding, had a few patients in the hospital. In the three months I was there I managed to spend one evening only in Auckland. Once I admitted to the hospital a VAD with a pleural effusion. I was half-way through aspirating her chest when Colonel Tewsley (A.D.M.S.) paid a surprise visit. He was horrified at my intrepidity and swept the girl into the Auckland Hospital almost before I had time to remove the needle.

There was enough time for rueful reflection. I had become a sort of military general practitioner: two field ambulances, a training school, a general hospital, a con. depot and now an S.M.O. To say nothing of having once been a lance corporal. The conviction grew on me that Wellington had forgotten that I was in Papakura. Kalavere, I heard, had been abandoned and the buildings were about to fall before the bulldozers. I began to compose a letter to General Bowerbank. Before I could get it on paper, General Bowerbank wrote to me, a blunt notification that I had been appointed O.C. Troops on the N.Z. Hospital Ship *Maunganui*.

After twenty-four perplexed hours I wrote back. I did not refuse – that cannot be done in the army – but with enormous respect I questioned the wisdom of his choice. I knew nothing of the navy, I had never even seen a hospital ship, I was utterly ignorant of its administrative routine . . . . It was so convincing that I felt a little contrite at the predicament in which I was now placing him and I added, 'Despite all this if it is your express wish that I should be appointed to this command . . . .' The reply was prompt. 'It is my express wish that you take over this command. You will proceed immediately on ten days' leave and will report to the ship on [date given] and will sail two days later.'

I left Papakura unwept and unweeping. The C.O. of the camp, who had been for a long time vainly trying to go overseas, regarded my appointment as a personal slight, especially as it left him in charge of a camp that could not now boast a single medical officer. We had never been close friends and our parting (which interrupted his composition of a stern letter to Wellington) was brief and chilly. I could have been a scapegoat driven out into the wilderness had it not been for a sloppy salute from my driver as he deposited me at the station.

At Wellington I applied confidently to the Railway Transport officer, Major Gentry, for a booking on the ferry that night. He had none – not even a shakedown, not even a few square feet of deck space. Not a possible vacancy under ten days – rank, urgency of mission notwithstanding. Planes? The plane situation was worse. But he was famed for his help to stranded soldiers. He dismissed me with the comment, 'Pity you weren't airforce. There's a service plane leaving for Wigram today at 1200 hours. But strictly airforce of course.'

I went out to the airport. A likely looking plane stood afar off. In due course nearly a dozen blue-clad figures strolled across the tarmac and embarked. I followed and took a rear seat. 'This the plane for Wigram?' I asked the nearest man. He nodded. The Air Force has always been inclined to overlook the Army. This time they overlooked me. No further word was spoken. It was a smooth trip. At Wigram I was saluted by the guard at the gate.

10

The Great White Lady

I arrived in Wellington on the appropriate date and reported at Army Headquarters about mid-morning and was coolly greeted by a trio of the Headquarters' staff. Where had I been? They had been waiting an hour. I was pushed into a car and rushed to the ship. There was a throng of brass and braid on the foredeck, General Bowerbank, Captain Prosser, Master of the ship, officials of the Union Steamship Company, the chief engineer and others of vague identity. There were also two lifeboats newly fitted with marine engines. Apparently I had to be convinced that the engines were strong enough. But why me? Surely the Master . . . . Yes, the Master if they were to be reserved for shipwrecks. Instead they were for the transport of patients. The engines were started. The din was dreadful, even alarming. If there was any correlation between noise and power, then I was satisfied. I looked interrogatively at Captain Prosser. He nodded. I looked at the chief engineer. He too nodded. In a short time everyone was nodding. So I nodded too and immediately the engines were stopped. There was a burst of conversation as I signed some forms and the boats were taken on charge. The group broke up. Someone said to me, 'Now sir, would you like to see over the ship?' I ceased to be a marine engineer (permanently) and became an apprehensive O.C. Troops.

I saw over the ship, going passively where I was led. To my noncritical eye she was enormous (about seven thousand five hundred tons, or twice the weight of an inter-island ferry). She had been a transport in the first war, a luxury liner thereafter and now was a hospital ship. The conversion had involved painting the ship white, adding four red crosses; tearing out the lounge fittings and filling the space with beds; sweeping out the cabins and so creating hospital wards, of which there was a total of eleven. There was also an orderly room, an X-ray plant, a change room, an operating theatre, a dispensary, a locked psychiatric ward, and an occupational therapy resort. On the boat deck the cabins were for officers on one side and on the other for Sisters and VADs.

It was essentially an army unit, with uniform, rank, parades, military discipline and daily routine orders. It was the only unit that was directly

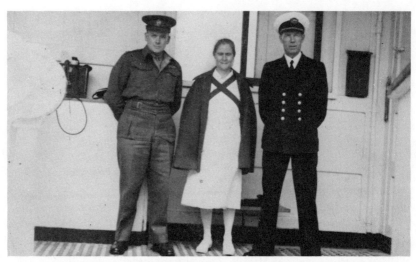

O.C. Troops, Matron and Master, H.M.N.Z.H.S. *Maunganui*

under the command of N.Z.A.H.Q. Wellington gave us our orders though in foreign ports we came partly under the control of the local officials. But in effect the further we were from Wellington the greater was our autonomy and also our efficiency.

On the ship itself authority came from two sources only, the Master and the O.C. Troops. Each had his sphere. Everything belonging to the ship, its safety, maintenance and manipulation as well as the control of the crew in all matters other than health was the responsibility of the Master. The O.C. Troops had under his command his staff of one hundred and four, his three hundred or more patients and a duty to ensure at all times the maximum medical efficiency.

It was a foolproof system. Neither Captain Prosser nor I wished to invade the other's territory and to struggle with the other's technicalities. In any impasse the deciding factor was the safety of the ship and here the Master was supreme. The O.C. Troops could request a certain line of action in the interests of patients. The Master would agree unless the safety of the ship was involved. Then his decision was final.

Despite such a simple formula for control it was not always accepted in the first war, and there were even conflicts in the second war. I once visited another hospital ship in Leyte Gulf. As I returned Captain Prosser paused at the head of the gangway and said, 'Well, how are things going over there?' 'Smoking and smouldering. There's a furious interchange of offensive notes. The O.C. Troops is going to put a message through to Whitehall if the Master does not apologize by 1400 hours.'

'Good Lord.' He took me by the elbow. 'Come and have a drink.'

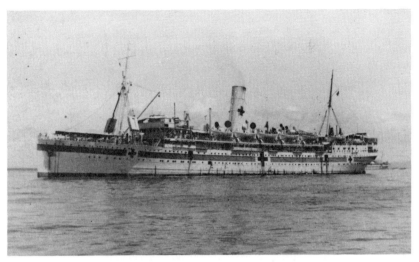

'The Great White Lady', H.M.N.Z.H.S. *Maunganui*

In retrospect, the success of the ship – and let it be said now, openly and defiantly, that it was highly successful – largely centred on the personality of Captain Prosser. He had all the medical interests deeply at heart. He mixed with us in a social role in the lounge and knew personally large numbers of the staff. He and I daily inspected the quarters of staff and crew. We found little to criticize. His predecessor and mine had set a high standard and almost always it was maintained.

To the Sisters, Captain Prosser was a kind of father figure. They teased him, played practical jokes on him but always at a level that left his authority and dignity wholly intact. His nautical cap was never worn to the saloon. If he hung it up for a moment he would have to recover it from the head of some Sister strutting the deck. His exit from the supper table was at least once impeded by his shoe laces being tied round the legs of the table. One day after ship's inspection he took me down to the paint room in the bow. The ship was rising and falling. The air was thick with oil and turpentine and lack of oxygen. He produced two black oily cigars and for fifteen minutes we smoked in the dark and in silence. This, I knew, was my examination for the certificate of sea-worthiness. Those who passed where those who at the end of the period showed no alteration of colour in their faces. As we reached the light of day and he turned me round I got in first with the phrase I had rehearsed in the paint locker, 'I say, you don't look too good'. He was surprised at my audacity. But at the same time I had blunted his weapon. I got my certificate, a treasured acquisition even though it was only verbal.

Prominent among the officers was Major Hugh Stevely, the Adjutant and 2 I/C (now an obstetrician of Dunedin). He was a veteran of many voyages and every refinement of administration was known to him. Of all his excellent qualities the one I appreciated most was his loyal co-operation in teaching me my job. In each of our ports of call a strict procedure had been laid down by the port authorities. I was quite prepared to do in Rome as the Romans did if only I knew what they also did in Fremantle, Colombo, Bombay, Aden, Tewfik, Port Said and Bari. With Major Stevely as my tutor, I learned it all in one voyage. He in turn was ably assisted by the R.S.M. (Regimental Sergeant-Major), Alan Gilkinson (later managing director of NAC).

A valued asset to the unit was Captain Jock Allen, paymaster and duty officer. I was never quite sure what this latter meant but it mattered little for he was indefatigable in his interpretation of it. Anything that contributed to the welfare of patients or staff, to entertainment, or to improving morale immediately commanded his interests and his activities. In later years, at ship's reunions, his ebullience had not slackened. At the end of the war he was strongly recommended for a decoration but owing to an administrative bungle (not on the ship) he did not receive it. His able assistant was Sergeant Norman Balfour (now an executive of Dalgety Loan in Napier).

The Quartermaster was Captain H. Broome. His was an exacting task. The ship has to sail adequately equipped with everything from buttons, needle and thread to the concrete blocks for weighting bodies buried at sea. I never heard of any reasonable request which Captain Broome could not supply.

The Matron was Miss Thwaites who, like me, was on her first voyage and like me, was feeling her way. She smoothly regulated the female staff. Her predecessor, Miss Lewis ('Mum') was, in my day, a legend. No one could tell me why in clear terms, but this was presumably because personality is hard to describe. My informants all mentioned her black dressing gown, her vigilance in the dark corners of the ship at night, her rigid rejection of an unstable story and her general popularity.

The senior physician on my first voyage was an old friend, Charles Burns (now Sir Charles Burns). He was a dedicated clinician and a dedicated teacher and inevitably before long he had organized clinics among the junior medical officers. These, along with dental officers, were often merely passengers to the Middle East. In that their journey by hospital ship freed more beds in transports for combatants, their presence with us was of doubtful legality. Our padres were Bishop Girard who had been senior chaplain in Necal and Father Martin who ministered to the Roman Catholics.

198

It is impossible to deal with the Sisters, VADs and O/Rs in other than general terms. Sister Kerr, Sister Haworth and Quartermaster Sergeant Scully had embarked on the first voyage. They all formed a harmonious team and had to. Anyone unhappy on board could get transferred on application. At the end of each voyage the O.C. Troops could submit a list to Army Headquarters of those whom he would like replaced. He did not have to give reasons and invariably his requests were granted.

On the outward voyage to the Middle East the ship usually left Wellington almost empty. A few patients might be found at Fremantle, many more at Colombo and thereafter the ship would probably be full. This was because N.Z.A.H.Q. had offered our services to all Allied soldiers travelling north. The outward voyage was at first a leisurely one. The wards were painted where necessary; all the bedding, dressings and medical equipment was moved in. Plastic bandages were made and stockpiled. The customary ball was held on deck when the tropics were reached. Maximal leave was granted at every port. Soon would come the demands of over three hundred sick soldiers homeward bound.

This was the *Maunganui*, a ship built round a dedicated staff, which was always zealous of its continuing good name. I had come among them an unknown and ignorant landlubber. There would have been full justification for a certain aloofness till I had proved myself. Instead I was welcomed and my authority fully recognized. Through them my transformation into a sailor was accelerated and in time I think I led them all in pride of the ship and its staff.

After a storm in the Tasman in which no one was sick or even dared to be sick if he wished to stay on the staff, we were welcomed by the Perth Red Cross. Their generosity was the same as I had experienced twenty-five years before. The special bonds between the ship and the Red Cross survived long after the war, so that at subsequent reunions of the ship's staff a cablegram of felicitations was usually received from Perth.

A new broom must be cautiously used. It was the custom for those O/Rs not on duty to parade every morning in battledress. On the wind-swept and rolling deck they attempted drill movements among the capstans, ring bolts and ropes. I abolished this farce to the joy of the troops.

A ship's magazine (*Whatknots*) was started with no editorial policy beyond promoting the welfare and the amusement of all on board. The standard edition was of four cyclostyled foolscap sheets. Everyone received a copy and anyone could contribute. And I, as editor, was surprised at the large number who did, including some members of the crew. It was also surprising how some stolid types could embark on imaginative flights of invention and fancy.

The ship had to be fuelled every ten days. And so we came to Colombo and its special feature of a warm wind lifting off the unwashed streets. What a riot of colour there is in the tropics! Here too was that Middle East phenomenon indigenous to all the ports of call, the furtive thrusting itinerant traders usually hawking magnificent solitaire diamonds reduced from a colossal sum to a few rupees, 'just for you'.

Bombay, gateway to India, was where the spies of the Allies and the Axis met and the tightest security controlled the wharves. It was impossible to land without a standard leave pass. We had none on board nor could they be procured elsewhere than on shore. It was made quite plain by the staff that the matter of passes was my concern. So I went ashore with Captain Prosser, who had an international pass. While he deliberately engaged the attention of the guard I slipped behind him. It nearly succeeded but another guard casually asked to see my pass and was suddenly alerted and blew a whistle. A noisy Indian crowd gathered, and though unaware of the matter in hand they abused the police and supported me. But the police won. In a police car I reached police headquarters. After a while I convinced them that I was not a master spy ingeniously disguised.

I was passed on to a British organization which I could not identify. It was presided over by a tall Englishman, lean, tanned, moustached, a true Kipling sahib. He commiserated with me. Yes, the situation was ridiculous, but security often threw up such situations. His office might have a few passes but had no authority to issue them. He got up and walked up and down. If I liked he would apply on my behalf for an issue of passes. It would take about a week. He looked out the window, his back to me. It was then I saw on the corner of his table a book of one hundred leave passes, where they certainly had not been a few moments before. I said we would be going in a few days. He turned round to a bare table. We digressed to the political situation of India, and disposed of it in less than a minute. We parted very good friends bound by the best of British traditions. His last admonition was that if ever I did get any of these elusive leave passes I would be wise to forget where I got them.

The next day all available staff were on shore. I followed. The Indian guard gave one glance at the signature on my pass and, not knowing it was mine, confidently waved me on.

At Tewfik there was much activity. Some passengers left, including Major Burns. New Zealand troops swarmed aboard, officials with papers and non-officials seeking a lettuce or an apple or even a bit of home gossip. I had business in Cairo and on my only day there saw the Tutankhamun treasures in the Cairo museum, on their first day of public exhibition.

Back at Tewfik we had embarked over two hundred Yugoslav partisans, male and female, veteran guerrilla fighters. They were fiercely independent, mistrusting any friendly advances and insisting on retaining their rifles and grenades under their pillows. How was I to equate this with the Geneva Convention? The mailed fist or the blind eye? I used the mailed fist in theory and the blind eye in practice. They kept to themselves and moved everywhere as a solid phalanx even on to a patch of deck which they appropriated and where they lustily sang their patriotic songs. This was outside the cabin of the chief steward who worked most of the night and slept part of the day. He would erupt, shaking his fist or shouting abuse. This they interpreted as a fiery approval and it always inspired them to an encore.

We could not communicate with them for we had no common tongue. Yet every day they took a copy of routine orders and typed out their version of it. They would crowd round and, as one read it out, they would sometimes roar with laughter. On every copy was my name and the name of the ship as if guaranteeing the veracity of the rest.

In the Mediterranean their mood changed. They stayed below, were sullen and unfriendly. Something was brewing and it had to be stopped. How important is speech. Then someone suggested a certain orderly, a private who was brilliant at miming and burlesque. He had even made the Yugoslavs laugh. They in turn had tried to teach him their language but he had got only as far as the Yugoslav word for 'good' which (I think) was *dobra*. This seemed neither adequate nor appropriate to launch an enquiry into something that presumably was bad. Yet he was sent below. The word was overworked but with it went a profusion of grimaces and gestures and inflexions. He was suddenly fluent in the truly international language of signs. They crowded round. The air was thick with noise and *dobras*. At length he reported confidently to me that there were five complaints which he enumerated. They were all minor and easily adjusted. Yugoslavs went back to the decks again, singing, presumably, the victor's hymn. We shed them at Taranto and the only ceremony was a certain amount of verbal exchange. We hoped they were expressing thanks. They probably assumed that we were wishing them well as indeed we were. We were wishing them a safe journey home across the Adriatic and a long stay there.

As they moved down the gangway at Taranto the staff moved into the wards putting the final touches for the mass embarkation of the morrow. I had no part in this except to know the plan. It was a perfected drill long before my time. No unit is a good unit unless the officer in command can stand back and delegate authority. In any case I was wanted at a conference at Bari. I spent the night at 3 General Hospital. Early the next morning the long line of ambulances carrying three hundred and twenty three patients began to move out of Bari. The emotions of these men has been well described in the official history, *Medical Units of 2 N.Z.E.F. in Middle East and Italy* (War History Branch, Internal Affairs, Wellington 1952), pp. 407-8. They were elegantly prepared for embarkation, with notes fully written up, and the current treatment detailed, while the plaster casts had diagrams and instructions on the clean white surfaces.

I was detained in Taranto and arrived at Bari in the late morning. The Great White Lady, as the men called the ship, with her red crosses and green bands, stood out in that dingy harbour. To me it was always an emotional and proud moment to approach from land and see the ship again. The embarkation was nearly over when I arrived, a practiced exercise flawlessly perfected. I went through the wards, all full, all functioning smoothly. We had arrived with our Yugoslavs crowding the decks. In less than twenty-four hours we were out in the Mediterranean again with New Zealanders filling our wards.

The ship immediately became a hospital. Daily rounds by medical officers, daily dressings, plaster changes, some operations, 'shaping the stump' of the amputees, security in the psychiatric ward.

At Tewfik we acquired a few more patients and received last minute instructions. Here I was informed that the Governor of Suez was coming to pay his respects and that mine was the social responsibility. He arrived, an enormous gentleman in a dazzling uniform with an aide and an interpreter. They filled my cabin and quite outshone my drab khaki shirt and shorts. I opened with a comment on the weather but this revealed that the interpreter had not much more English than had the Yugoslavs. So I poured a round of whisky, the proven international loosener of tongues. In desperation we went back to the weather but I was misunderstood. I gathered that Egypt had no weather. Part of the time it was hot and for the rest of the time it was hotter. This meteorological truth justified another drink. I asked if he would like to see over the ship. He shook his head emphatically. He had probably misunderstood me again. I asked the meaning of Tewfik and the reply was voluble and incomprehensible. His Excellency seemed amused and helped himself. For a quarter of an hour we shuffled about bilingually and pseudo-bilingually. Officers with curious glances kept passing and repassing the open door of my cabin. Some of them I had invited to the party but they had all been too busy to come. At last His Excellency sat bolt upright and put his hands on his knees. Mentally I helped him to his feet. He said (I think) that he was very impressed with the ship which he had not seen. I said I was very impressed with Egypt despite the lack of weather. We parted with a cordiality primed by alcohol. The occasion, despite its restricted agenda, had been an international success.

There was mist and steam in the Red Sea, an oily film in the tropics, petulant seas in the south. The heat went out of the day and moisture out of the night. The ambulant became more ambulant and fresh faces kept appearing on deck. Occupational therapy (a special department under Miss Audsley Cullen) became a craze and Donald Ducks in extravagant disguises appeared all over the ship. A little list of seriously ill remained. There was an occasional burial at sea, in the grim dawn with the engines at half-speed and the officers standing by, and at the appropriate place in the padre's intonation the Quartermaster would lift one end of the board. There would be a movement under the flag and for a moment a darker shape on the face of the dim sea. The padre would conclude and the mourners melt away. The engines would pick up. The Master would record the position in nautical terms and transmit it to the Admiralty. A lightening eastern sky would announce another day and down in the diet kitchen the orderlies would start rattling their dixies.

When the Southern Cross came up there was a shift of interest from Italy to New Zealand. The Red Cross was waiting for us at Perth, generous as ever. But many of the ambulant patients were looking, not for Red Cross comforts, but for beer, cooled beer that they had dreamed about in the desert. And at Fremantle and Perth there was beer often forced on them by generous Australians. I had heard lugubrious tales of the consequences on previous voyages. It needed only two or three drunk men in Sister's immaculate ward to turn it into a shambles. How to prevent it? I rejected the stupid autocracy of refusing leave or putting all pubs out of bounds. Instead I preferred to let the men discipline themselves. So the day before we reached Fremantle I called a parade of those going on shore. I described what had happened on previous voyages, the débâcle in the wards and the set-back to the careful work of doctors and nurses. I appealed for a new deal. I asked for sobriety as a minimum and if possible on this special occasion, abstinence. I stressed that it was a request and not an order. It was an emotional appeal. It was meant to be. The time was ripe. They, more fortunate than thousands of others, were going to be back home in Wellington at the end of next week.

And it worked, despite the scepticism of some of my officers. They came back that night in little quiet groups. There was no noise, no shouting, no misbehaviour. A few were a little unsteady and some of these deliberately paraded in front of me repeatedly coming to attention but failing to maintain it. 'Thought yer orter see us, sir,' said one. 'Thought yer orter be proud of us.'

203

I was proud of them. I was more proud of them than I was of myself. The taste of victory was suddenly sour. They were freedom fighters, these men, and one of the freedoms was the right to a harmless skinful of beer. What right had I to go pussyfooting among their ideals? Still, I had helped the Sisters. I went round the wards late that night. Everyone slept. It was an improvement, agreed the Sisters the next day. But they had no enthusiasm for the improvement. None of them thanked me. It was clear that the men were still their patients, intemperate or not and, despite the consequences, their sympathies were more with the thirsty returning Kiwis than with a starry-eyed commanding officer.

How lovely is Wellington harbour when the engines sigh to a stop. How lovely is the city terraced over its hills. How lovely is the head of the harbour with spangles of light from the roofs of Petone and the purple obscurity of the Hutt Valley. A barge-load of officials – pilot, Army, Health Department, Harbour Board, Customs, press, government – swarmed on board. My cabin was so full I could hardly enter. The ship began to edge into a wharf packed with cheering people. The gangways went down and were almost immediately filled with patients, some on stretchers, some on crutches, some on foot. There was no attempt at an ordered disembarkation, which would be discipline only for the sake of discipline. There was an inevitable and excusable confusion on the wharf as kin met kin.

Then there was a drift to the Casualty Clearing Station. The Prime Minister, the Rt. Hon Peter Fraser, made a prim speech of welcome and received little attention. On behalf of the patients, the O.C. Troops made an even more prim reply and got even less attention. I went with General Bowerbank to confront the Adjutant-General, Brigadier Conway, to explain away my very liberal interpretation of certain orders. That done, I presented my demands – unit funds, a workshop, improved messing arrangements for convalescents. That night we sailed for Lyttelton where the South Island patients were carried to a hospital train. I had a few days in Christchurch, then went to Wellington. The ship was filling again with stores. Carpenters were busy on the projects I had sought. I spent a lot of time at A.H.Q.

We left on the fifteenth voyage carrying a large number of medical and dental officers to the Middle East. We had a splendid staff. The senior surgeon was the highly competent Major O'Regan from Wellington, hearty and affable and a natural shipmate. The senior physician was Major S. L. Ludbrooke of Auckland, quieter, no less loyal and sincere and a first-rate clinician. In the troubled days to come no better choice could have been made than of these two key officers.

We were four days from Fremantle. And in the early hours of the morning I was awakened by a message from the Master. We were being diverted to Melbourne. We were to join the British Pacific Fleet.

I was incredulous. There had been no hint of this at Wellington. The British Pacific Fleet was a mere name, known only to a few, and was not to be talked about. What had we to do with the fleet? I waited for an explanatory message from Wellington, but none ever came.

At Melbourne I had to abandon all suspicion that we were the victims of a mistake or even a hoax. Clearly we had to join the fleet. Where was the fleet? No one knew. And what did we do when we got there? No one knew. We discharged our few patients to hospitals. Our dental and medical passengers were marched off to a nearby camp. And we were sent to Sydney. At Sydney I asked the same question. Where and why? We were going to Manus, they said. And why? No one knew. It was obvious that the ship would acquire a new role. Were we suitably equipped? Majors Stevely, Ludbrooke, O'Regan and I considered all medical possibilities. We foresaw the likelihood of dysentery, typhus, malaria, wounds and burns. We might need large quantities of plasma. We made out a list. That afternoon Rear Admiral Fleet Train (R.A.F.T.) delivered it all by barge. An hour later we were *en route* to Manus.

Manus, chief of the Admiralties, is a humid island pegged to the equator like a damp sock on a clothes line. It is long, heavily jungled and from the sea is a milky blue arc on the horizon. It has, so it is said, a splendid natural harbour. We never saw it on any of our visits. The area was always too crowded with vessels.

We anchored far out. The Master and I were summoned on shore. We landed at a little barnacled jetty on a shingly beach. There had been a storm and the grey-green waves kept lunging at the sour and rotting terraces of dead jungle. Just beyond were the moving legions of ants and hermit crabs. Easily I could have been back on Vella Lavella. Manus, though British, was now American. We found the appropriate naval authorities and received the simple instructions that we were to proceed to the Philippines to join the British Pacific Fleet.

Gradually we learned of the British Pacific Fleet. It has been called the Unknown Fleet or the Forgotten Fleet. The secrecy surrounding it was at first deliberate, both to confuse the Japs and to preserve the American image in the Pacific. It was in fact the greatest concentration of naval power the British Navy has ever known. On V.J. Day it comprised four battleships, nine aircraft carriers with eight escorts, ten cruisers, forty destroyers, thirty submarines and a hundred and seventy six other vessels.

Very briefly, it may here be said that the British Fleet was of great importance in the war against Japan. It helped with final destruction of the Japanese navy, engaged the Japanese air forces repeatedly and bombed oil refineries, airfields and military targets from Malaya up to the mainland of Japan. It was not well equipped for the vast distances of the Pacific. The nearest base was Sydney, over four thousand miles from Japan. This meant that all the massive equipment necessary to keep a fleet operational had to travel with it in a fleet train. A new type of naval warfare resulted. There was no precedent for a floating fleet train of such magnitude. It was a matter of improvisation with necessity as a keynote. The result was truly international, the vessels coming from Britain, France, Norway, the Netherlands, Australia and New Zealand.

The Pacific portion of the fleet, as opposed to the East Indies portion, required six hospital ships. The first was the *Oxfordshire*, a British ship, very well equipped but strangely different from the *Maunganui*. We were the second ship, our Middle East run having been taken over by the *Oranje*. The *Tjitzalengka*, Mussolini's Mediterranean pleasure yacht, was the third hospital ship, but because of defective engines was making slow progress to the Pacific. At a later stage came the *Gerusalemme*. We made for the Philippines (where there are over seven thousand islands), through the Coral Sea and the Inland Philippine Sea, where the Americans had won the greatest naval victory of the war ('Trafalgar of the Pacific').

We anchored in Leyte Gulf, a white intruder among a vast array of dark shapes dotting the light blue sea. We exchanged courtesies with the flagship and with the *Oxfordshire*. Captain Curry, Senior Medical Officer of R.A.F.T., advised us of the details of our mission. We were to take such illnesses and wounds as were beyond the scope of their own ships. Our senior medical men were to act as consultants. He would expect us at all times to do anything we thought appropriate. Captain Curry was a good friend to us. Later when he himself fell ill he preferred to be admitted to our ship.

Immediately our routine was modified and the first problem was transport. Naval ships at sea are usually boarded by rope nets. So a landing stage, sturdy and capacious, was made by the ship's carpenter. It led by strong steps to a similar stage flush with the deck and was designed to bear stretchers. Few ships had their own small boats. Routine orders declared that our two powered boats were reserved solely for the transfer of patients, unless specially directed by the Master or O.C. Troops. Our signallers became invaluable. All day they would scan the sea for ships calling us up. Our orderlies became expert gangway stretcher-bearers. Occasionally a fighting ship would arrive with a long list of wounded. The theatre lights would go on, the plasma drips be set up, and Major O'Regan would decide his priorities. We had a naval liaison warrant officer. We adapted to naval terms, naval adminstration, naval thinking.

The ship became well and favourably known. The personality of the Sisters was a major factor in this. So also was the clinical ability of Majors O'Regan and Ludbrooke, the perfected administration of Major Stevely and the felicitous personality of the indefatigable Captain Allen. We held clinical meetings, which were well attended by medical officers from nearby ships, including the consulting surgeon to the fleet, Professor Lambert Rogers of Cardiff. We persisted with every kind of activity we knew. The ship swung idly round its anchor and the monotony streamed in every morning with the heat. There was no leave.

Some minor adventures involved the nursing staff. A curious friendship developed between some Norwegian ratings and some Sisters. Neither knew a word of the others' tongue. They were middle-aged homely men. Every week or so their noisy little boat would chug up to our landing stage and embark five or six nurses. In their fo'c'sle they would sit around, the Sisters darning socks and patching garments, while the men passed round photos of their families. All the time there would be an animated conversation by means of gestures, mime, facial expression, inflexions on English or Norwegian words, or subtle variations of laughter. Then would come an elaborate supper and soon they would be going down one gangway and then up another.

Less engaging was the approach of an American, captain of an engineer's supply ship. He was lively, amusing, generous and persistent. He was a frequent visitor, specially when nurses were off duty. I suspected he had some plan in mind and that it was first necessary to soften me up. He implied deep friendship and offered us all the engineering resources of America. He was full of admiration for our occupational therapy. Then he discovered that I had no toolset of my own and came back the same day with some chisels and a vice; I have them still. I played along, warily. When he must have considered me ripe for a picking he informed me that he had just had a brilliant idea. The idea of a moonlight picnic. He and half a dozen or so of his fellow officers and an equal number of Sisters out on the placid sea under an enormous tropical moon wrapped in the mysterious essence of the night. There was a splendid beach on the Leyte mainland . . . . There would, he supposed airily, be no objection. I said the Sisters worked hard all day . . . . Yes, he knew that, but a moonlight picnic was so magical, so invigorating . . . . Confidently he left me to think it over. I asked Matron. She looked startled and shook her head. He came back. I suggested he make it a daylight picnic and Matron and I could come too. To his credit he showed nothing of the horror he must have felt.

207

His next move was to invite me out in his launch. We would land south of Tacloban. And this we did. It was a beautiful launch. The land was dry and dusty, covered with a thorny scrub in which were a few miserable shacks. Back in the boat he produced the whisky again and kept the bottle hovering over my paper cup. As a point of discussion he sought my opinion on the greatest man in the present war. I said Roosevelt. He disagreed. It was Churchill. Obviously the attack was now on. He filled my cup again. I think I might like whisky if someone would invent a method of changing the taste. Most of what he gave me went unobtrusively into the Philippine Sea. Then I saw that he was doing the same. Somehow we shared the knowledge and his adventure lost momentum. He took me back to the ship, dropped me at the gangway and chugged off. He returned to the subject on other occasions but without much hope. Had he known how small his chances had ever been he would not have wasted a bottle of lemonade on me.

The fleet came back, not in orderly convoy but in scattered units over several days till all round us were the spreading immensities of the carriers, the towering superstructure of the battleships, the sweeping lines of the cruisers. We were dwarfed, but not in spirit. This was the navy and we were part of it, as had been Raleigh and Drake and Nelson.

Then came V.E. Day. We received from Whitehall the traditional naval message that marks special occasions: 'Splice the mainbrace' (Serve rum ration to all hands); 'Deck ship, fore and aft' (display all the bunting available); and 'make and mend' (once a period reserved for repairing clothing, but later synonymous with a general holiday). We got out our lifeboats and competed regatta-like with the *Achilles* and in the evening held a dance. But we had none of the roaring jubilation of Europe. We were still at war and V.E. Day belonged to another war. Our war was in the Pacific and was not aimed at the occupation of Berlin, but at the revenge of Pearl Harbour.

At length there came the expected order. The fleet was to return to Sydney in the interests of oil, water, stores and morale. Most of our patients went back to their own ships. We sailed on 21 May. The *Oxfordshire* followed three days later. The *Tjitzalengka*, because of its better supplies, stayed at Leyte.

The fleet had arrived when we reached Sydney, crowding the great harbour even to the little bays. Waiting for us was the New Zealand Liaison Officer determined to refute a rumour that his job was not necessary. He brought with him a telephone already connected. In the crowded convalescent patients' mess he welcomed us to what he understood was to be three weeks in Sydney. We would have a royal time in Sydney. He rattled off its attractions just as a guide would; would all those who would like a trip to the Blue Mountains signify . . .? A forest of hands rose. This was my moment to intervene. I had just been handed a message from the Master that we were sailing for New Zealand in fifteen minutes. We reversed the hospitality and gave him a drink. As the hawsers were cast loose and we slipped out in the harbour he almost failed to get ashore. He had to abandon the telephone. The wire was played out to the limit at both ends and eventually broke in the middle. Someone in New Zealand probably still has it (illegally).

Wellington hardly noticed us. There were a couple of ambulances on the wharf for our few patients, a few officials, a few relatives of staff. I went to A.H.Q. where all priority was now being given to men returning from the Middle East. I went round shaking hands. 'Been having great adventures they tell me,' said various ones. 'I must hear all about it.' And passed on rapidly in case I took them up. It was the shortest of leaves. All the staff had a day or two at home while the ship was replenished. And soon we were at sea again.

Manus was sweltering. The breeze would be cooler when we got to Leyte. Then we learned we were not going to Leyte. The *Tjitzalengka* was there. The *Oxfordshire* was in Sydney. The fleet train was building up at Manus. There were rumours of an attack on Singapore and a linking with the East Indies half of the fleet. We were very necessary at Manus. So we let down the gangway, and men and messages began to flow.

There followed a miserable period redeemed only by the fact that we had plenty to do and by all accounts did it well. But the ship swung slowly on its anchor in the blast of the day and the velvety moisture of the night. The island was a faint blur, miles away, and nearer were only a few coral strips supporting a drunken palm or two. Bathing was impossible because of sharks. All diversionary interests were exploited, but the greatest of these was the quiz contest. It swept the ship, first with interest and then with excitement. Six teams – unit officers, Sisters, O/Rs and patients, merchant navy officers and stewards – entered. Every Thursday night another round was broadcast over the whole ship. Its popularity owed a very great deal to the personality of the Quizmaster, Major O'Regan. He would sit inflexible as a Buddha, restricting his amusement to a low rumble, indifferent to appeals or scorn. At one stage he had a senior Medical Officer squirming because he did not know what a caduceus was. He disarmed a steward with preliminary remarks on zoos and giraffes and then suddenly asked him what a carafe was. It was estimated he had filled at least ten a day for thirty years. But he hadn't called them carafes. That wasn't what he called them either in the next few weeks when he brooded over the tragedy. One erudite steward, who wrote a splendid feature for

Whatknots ('Pepys Diary'), was asked the difference between hamlet and omelette and defined them both as masterpieces, one by William Shakespeare, the other by John Shakespeare, which was the name of the ship's chief chef. What is frangipani, was one question. Frangipani was a tree growing in tropical countries. . . the details went on. Frangipani, said the Quizmaster, is a scent. The audience expostulated – but in vain. The telephone rang. Captain Prosser presented his compliments to Major O'Regan and begged to inform him that frangipani is a tree. Major O'Regan thanked Captain Prosser for his valued opinion and assured him that frangipani is the scent of red jasmine. Again the phone rang. Someone from the sacred regions forward intimated that Captain Prosser was on his way down. Captain Prosser appeared and took over. He discussed briefly the geography of the Pacific and his personal knowledge of its innumerable frangipani-studded ports. He established frangipani trees as one of the glories of the Pacific. At the end Major O'Regan, putting his hand on two massive dictionaries, 'Quite so, but frangipani is a scent.' Years later, O'Regan told me, he sat in a barber's chair in Wellington; the barber, a stranger, adjusted the towel and said: 'Tell me, what is frangipani?'

One of our difficulties was lack of boats for recreation. Even to fish near the reef would have been something. Lying not far away was the aircraft carrier *Illustrious*, damaged and about to leave for England, and it carried some fourteen foot sailing dinghies, recreational craft only. One of these we coveted. The approach was difficult. After all we were only an army unit. But, pressured by my officers, I had to do something.

'To the Boat Officer. Please inform conditions on which we might acquire one of your sailing dinghies?'

Within a few minutes came the reply, 'On condition the vessel is sailed away by an entirely female crew'.

'Generous terms approved. Please advise appropriate time for transfer. E.F.C. in training.'

'Tomorrow 1530.'

I then laid the signals before Matron who was appalled. None of her girls knew anything about yachts. . . but she was wrong. One of the Sisters was a keen yachtswoman. Two others had been forced to mess about in boats by older brothers. A fourth was keen to learn. So the team was fixed, (Sisters Mary Noonan and Boh Webster, and VADs Gwen Leonard and Merle Ridley). Till late that evening they were quartered with Major Ludbrooke being instructed in the secret life of yachts. They left amid cheers in one of our powered boats manned by two of the marine officers and captained by Major Ludbrooke. At the landing stage of the *Illustrious* they were helped off by a waiting officer who led them up the gangway. Discreetly our officers attempted to follow but were politely sent back. Our emissaries disappeared, presumably for the benefit of afternoon tea. Within an hour they re-appeared surrounded by a cluster of officers. Far below was the dinghy moored by a rope to the end of a boom. Then there were signs that the party was breaking up. And suddenly, dramatically, it did. The leader of our quartette shuffled out along the boom, shinned down the rope and into the dinghy. The rest followed. They did various things to the sails (I am no yachtsman) and drifted off. The aircraft carrier cheered. We cheered. The cheering, I was informed later, was at the prodigious feat of manning the dinghy from the boom. It showed impeccable manners by champion yachtsmen. Four members of the N.Z. Army Nursing Service were not supposed ever to have heard of it, let alone have the skill and the courage to perform it. It was a splendid and valuable dinghy. The Quartermaster who was heading up a form to take it on charge was warned off. It was made very plain in *Whatknots* that it belonged to the personnel of the unit. By popular vote it was taken to Wellington (Captain Prosser gave it deck space) and was given to the R.N.Z. Volunteer Naval Reserve training depot, to be used solely for the recreation of ratings.

A message came one day that a sick English officer on an island about one hundred miles away required medical attention. Major Ludbrooke and I were ordered to investigate. We flew in a three-seater plane with a dual cockpit. We saw not only our patient, whose state was not alarming, but an American hospital with a pharmacist's mate in charge. He had fifty patients in bed all suffering, he said confidently, from scrub typhus. He may have been right and if so then a century of diagnosis of scarlet fever in New Zealand has been wrong.

On the return journey we changed pilots and also seats in our little metallic sandfly. Major Ludbrooke occupied the gunner's seat behind while I sat next the pilot, a boisterous extrovert who poured scorn on the craft, said it was impossible to fly and took an affected farewell of his mates. When we were airborne he was amazed to learn that I could not fly. He insisted that I correct this immediately. He demonstrated the foot and hand controls and after a little practice I nodded to him confidently, whereupon he folded his arms, slipped down in his seat and appeared to sleep heavily. I flew on, savouring the magnificence of it all. The day was perfect. Far below was the green carpet of the sea, and above was the blue ceiling where the stars were pinned at night, and in between was I, in charge of a flying rat-trap. In effect I was flying solo, which must have been a record after a total of instruction estimated at four and a half minutes. I had gentle adventures with curious little wisps of cloud that came drifting up. At length, far off, I could see the white runway on the tiny island of our destination. The crazy thought came to me that it wouldn't really be difficult to bring her in and land. . . . At this moment the engine stopped. The plane plummeted sickeningly. The pilot sprang at the controls, restarted the engine, and woke up afterwards. Between us we probably set a world record for speed of change of control. Two records on one's first training flight is almost in itself a third record.

Suddenly, V.J. Day.

It was my third armistice on active service and this was the maddest of them all. There was an explosion of American exuberance which soon became American irresponsibility. Pearl Harbour had been avenged. A few days before, the last of the Japanese navy, fuelless and helpless, had been sunk in Japanese harbours. Retribution could go no further.

Communal rejoicing is usually compounded of noise and movement and little else. Every noisy contraption on every ship exploded into sound. Dozens of small boats appeared, crazily dashing from ship to ship. A favourite sport was to race broadside on to a ship and at the last moment put the helm hard over. As the boat slewed round the man on the stern might be thrown overboard, his life then depending on his sobriety. We heard grim stories later of the number of men so lost, all victims of victory. The American navy is dry, which is not to say it cannot occasionally get very wet.

We received the traditional signal again, 'Dress ship, fore and aft. Splice the mainbrace. Make and mend.' We were told that this was only the sixth occasion in this century when the order to splice the mainbrace had been made. For an army unit to receive such an order twice in the one year would probably be an enduring record. The rum was supplied in earthenware jars inside a basket frame. At dinner that night Major O'Regan and his surgical team were absent in the theatre. The previous evening we had embarked the victims of a kamikaze (suicide bomber) and on V.J. Day over thirty operations were performed. The rum ration for those in the theatre was estimated by shaking the container. It was a quantity more generous than wise and the consequences in no way conflicted with the levity of the day.

After dinner some of us at the Master's invitation went up on the bridge. It was a soft velvety night heavy with the tropics. Every ship was lit. They stretched to the horizon. Much of the British fleet, more of the fleet train, and vastly more of American vessels. The sky was ablaze with searchlights, rockets, star shells, tracer ammunition and a wide range of pyrotechnic substitutes. It was unorganized, undisciplined, garish, yet beautiful. Far off, Manus itself blazed with light, part of which came from the burning of the canteen.

We could not stand aloof. Captain Prosser found a number of old distress signals overdue for replacement. With them we added our modest quota to the display. At the very height of the colour and the clamour there came a general signal from the Island Command to all units ashore and afloat. It was an order to stop this night pageantry immediately.

Alas for the Island Command. He was an unpopular American whose name no one knew. He apparently believed that a whim or a precaution if dressed up as an order will divert a man from his compulsive instincts. No ship obeyed the signal and after a dutiful pause we resumed. But I was uneasy. Only a ship separated us from the *Montclare*, the flagship of Admiral Fisher. I had been his guest at dinner a few nights before, the only khaki figure there. He and his staff were charming hosts but I felt that we were with the fleet by grace and favour only.

Two days later I received an order to report to the Admiral at 0900 hours. I went with some apprehension. But he could not have been more affable. He discussed the future. Every urgency now had to be given to the repatriation of P.O.W.s. A British task force was moving into Hong Kong where there were two camps for internees. A number of the inmates could not be shifted except by hospital ship. The ship that went in would have to be readily adaptable to deal with an unknown number of unknown diagnoses. Resource and initiative would be required. Could we do it? Most emphatically we could do it. He nodded and proceeded to details. He would move the *Oxfordshire* up (then ten miles away) and it would take all our patients. A radio telephone would be installed on each ship so that I could discuss with the O.C. Troops *Oxfordshire* the details of the transfer. We would arrive in Hong Kong after the task force as certain organization was first necessary. The Master would receive appropriate instructions.

'All clear, Colonel?'

'Yes sir, quite clear.'

I got up to go. At the door of the stateroom I turned and saluted. Instead of acknowledging it he said,

'Just a minute, I'm curious about another little matter.' I went back.

'On your ship the other night were you firing off rockets?'

'I believe we did fire some.'

'And did you receive a message from the Island Command to stop?'

'Yes, I understand there was a message to that effect, sir.'

'And did you stop?'

'Oh yes, sir.'

'And then resume?'

'Well. . . .'

'Tell me. Did you, yourself, fire any rockets after that signal was received?'

'Yes, sir, I did.' There was a little pause. Then he said with emphasis,

'Good show, Bennett. Good show. So did I. The damned impertinence of the fellow.'

And so we left Manus and without regret. We came to Leyte Gulf again and as we dropped anchor our artist of the moonlight picnic came streaking across the water. His theme was the same but it was now a tired refrain. That night the moonlight was again wasted. We then anchored in Subic Bay, a grim battlefield. So was Corregidor, though little of this could be seen from the sea. Manila harbour was studded with the masts of sunken vessels. On the waterfront only one building (which may have been the Customhouse) remained intact. We were at the wharf for only a few hours. Most of the male staff were on shore in small groups for twenty minutes at a time. It allowed them to add another item to their geographic souvenirs. Twenty minutes was long enough. There was nowhere to go and nothing to see but devastation. The main street at the end of the wharf was completly blocked by a mountain of rubble.

Admiral Harcourt with Task Force 111.3 entered Hong Kong harbour on 30 August. His flagship was the cruiser *Swiftsure*. With him was the cruiser *Euryalus*, the destroyers *Tuscan* and *Kempenfelt*, and the auxiliary anti-aircraft ship *Prince Robert*. There were also submarines and mine sweepers. Outside the harbour in safe deep water were *Indomitable, Anson, Maidstone* and more destroyers and submarines. It must have been an emotional moment for the British civilian internees of Stanley Camp high up on the hill as the ships of the British Navy steamed through the narrow entrance and filled out the harbour. Some suicidal Japanese naval craft came out to battle. Aircraft from *Indomitable* sank them all.

In due course the *Maunganui* followed and berthed at one of the wharves of Kowloon on the mainland. My first impression of Hong Kong and my abiding impression to this day was of people. They massed everywhere on sea and land. Though in the last four years the Japanese had fulfilled their threat of reducing the population by two thirds, yet over half a million remained. Within twenty-four hours of the British arrival, and partly due to a civil administration set up by one of the ex-prisoners, Mr F. C. Gimson, a pre-war colonial secretary to the Hong Kong Government, all the Japs had been shifted from Victoria Island, which is Hong Kong proper, to the mainland of Kowloon. They needed little urging, for on the island they would have been inexorably exterminated by the Chinese. At Kowloon they had some protection. They were even ordered by the navy to mount guard over some selected buildings to prevent looting. One day I went down the main street in Kowloon and two naval ratings on guard presented arms. I saluted. At the next building two Japanese guards attempted the same movement and grotesquely bungled it. Should I have saluted? Anyhow I did.

The Allies defeated the Jap, but never understood him. It is said that a group of about forty pilots of suicide bombers, having had their funeral orations read and being, so to speak, dead except for the triviality of crashing on a target, had this blocked by the intervention of the armistice. This to a New Zealander would be making the best of two worlds – a hero in principle and an escapee in fact. But these Japanese took off and one by one dived into the sea, craft and all. In Hong Kong their new philosophy was that now the dreadful war was over we could all be friends. They seemed to imply that all combatants had been caught up helplessly in the disaster of war.

The Chinese had noisily and brutally repossesed Victoria Island. Crackers, fireworks, rockets continued day and night. Mixed with it all was an occasional rifle shot which no wise man would wish to investigate. The narrow streets were festooned with flags and bunting, and up and down, ceaselessly and apparently aimlessly, went the moving masses.

Less aimlessly moved the masses on the water. As we came opposite Kowloon the sampans rushed us from all quarters with women paddling furiously. They circled the ship begging, begging, begging. . . . These were the 'river Chinks', living on the scavengings of the harbour, living and dying on their sampans, denied education, pleasures, culture, aiming only at enough food for survival. At every meal on the ship the long bamboo rods bearing at the end their little string baskets would come through the portholes and hover over the tables in mute appeal for a crust or a scrap. There is a special ugliness about hunger in the mass. Life becomes cheapened. For our first twenty-four hours in Kowloon there were two dead Chinamen at the end of the wharf. In a busy Hong Kong street a nearly naked youth lay across the pavement, his body arched back in the last stages of meningitis while everyone (myself included) stepped over him. Funerals – typified by a barefoot coolie running along a street with a coffin on a rickshaw – were frequent and wasted nothing on the dead. In the sampans it was common to see listless children with abdomens distended with malaria or tuberculosis. Or it could have been malnutrition, for to the Jap this was a weapon of war, easy, economical and lethal. But the Chinese in turn had weapons of their own. One day I saw a Chinese barge crushed in the centre of an armada of sampans. In what appeared to be their thousands the people shouted and cheered, and launched the inevitable fireworks. The occasion was the keel-hauling of the Japanese harbour master. I did what I could for him – I wished that his death might be quick.

The civilian prisoners in Stanley Camp on Mt. Victoria had been liberated by Admiral Harcourt himself. Many of them came to us. The other camp was Shamsuipo for military P.O.W.s at Kowloon. Major Ludbrooke and I had a typical famine meal there, being their first and last guests. We planned with them the embarkation of their sick.

Of the apparent total of four cars in Kowloon one of them was acquired for our ship by some of the enterprising N.C.O.s using methods which I preferred not to have explained. It had 'Medical Officer of Health' across the windscreen. This was regarded by Admiral Harcourt as highly appropriate and he confirmed it in a light moment by appointing me M.O.H. for Hong Kong. The appointment was verbal only, and so would now be hard to prove. But it was legal within the sweeping powers given to him and, as far as I know, it still stands. The car was full of whims but one of the ship's officers was a specialist in crossed wires beneath dashboards. In it the nursing staff went in relays to a nearby Catholic convent where they could see the city and trade the news of the occupation with the news of the world. The men went ashore in groups. The streets were still dangerous. The Chinese were opening up their shops and stocking up with goods of which the Japs had known nothing. They had no idea of values and generally preferred New Zealand currency because the pound note was larger than that of any other currency.

We began to admit patients. There were few of the desperately ill cases we had been led to expect. Desperately ill prisoners did not live long. Most were frail and feeble, vaguely unwell, and needing planned investigation.

Meanwhile, all along the China coast and down through the East Indies to Burma the rescue work went on. America had the resources. The planes would roar over the inland P.O.W. camps parachuting supplies, even up to all requirements for blood transfusions. Then the rescue force would smash its way in. The obsequious Japs would be swept aside and the internees loaded onto trucks and thence to ships all bound to the central camp at Manila.

One of the problems concerned Formosa, where were the worst internment camps. The prisoners worked under slave conditions and at the same time faced a Japanese campaign of extermination, a protracted Belsen of the East. A major camp was Kinkasaki on the north east coast. Here the British P.O.W.s worked in the copper mines under conditions of slavery, starvation, beatings, and disease with no medical facilities. In the camp at any time were only the survivors, a few hundreds of the indomitable ones. Thousands had died. With every death the camp commandant would rub his hands and say, 'Soon my cemetery will be full'. Perhaps they had never lost hope, because hope always trails the footsteps of life, but they had nothing with which to nourish it. Their guards gave them news: Japan was victorious on all fronts, their allies, the Russians, had seized the Suez Canal, Roosevelt was weeping over his shortage of soldiers, Mountbatten had deserted his troops. Escape was impossible. (Two Americans who escaped were brought back and publicly decapitated.) Rescue . . .? How could there be rescue? Then suddenly the Japs softened. The dreadful war was nearly over. Soon they would all be friends again. The work in the mines stopped. The food rations of a cup of rice a day and the green stew made of boiled chrysanthemum tops was slightly increased. All the prisoners were then given an injection of aneurin. (I saw some of the ampoules, marked 'Vitamin B mg 1 (strong)'; this, supposed to cope with the deficiencies of years, was about a third of a normal day's requirements.) Suddenly the American rescue party arrived, weighted with food and luxuries and cigarettes. There was some rough handling of the Japs. The rescued climbed on to the jeeps and trucks which then crashed through the roadless jungle to the beaches.

But not all. There remained nearly two hundred too ill to move, unable to stand or sit, moving inexorably towards death from chronic malnutrition or chronic infections. Two British medical officers, Captain G. Black and Captain Lewis, both P.O.W.s, stayed with them. They could do little except safeguard them from the Japs. Drugs were not enough. Only urgent hospital care could save these men, but there were no hospitals. The only route out was along the copper ore trail, a crazy twenty-five mile railway to Kuling in the north. But Kuling was only a name for a group of gutted buildings and a small harbour full of sunken vessels.

The circumstances became known in Hong Kong. It was unthinkable that these men should first be rescued and then abandoned, a tragic footnote to victory. Captain Prosser and I were called to a naval conference. Could we . . .? We could. We pledged the ship. It was a short conference. That evening a task force of four vessels slipped out past the rocky headlands of Hong Kong harbour: a cruiser, the *Bermuda*, under the command of Rear-Admiral Servaes, two destroyers, and H.M.N.Z.H.S. *Maunganui*.

By 9 September the ships were off Keelung Island. It was a grey, looming day and the wireless kept crackling with gale warnings from the north. Far out, a saturnine Jap pilot, conversant with the minefield, boarded the *Maunganui*. After a little while Captain Prosser relieved him, confident of a clear lane in the wake of the ship ahead. It was a wild coast, the sea being dotted with black rocks, white-splashed. The harbour entrance was narrow and the harbour small and scarred with wrecks. Enclosing it on three sides were strips of bombed and blackened buildings, the whole setting as incongruous as a faded garland on a corpse. It was eerie and ugly. The *Maunganui* tied up at Number Two pier. Opposite were low, olive-grey hills, barren except for rare clumps of trees. There were no comely shapes, no uplift of colour.

It could have been dangerous country. The ships represented the first of the victors. On the hills, a few chains away, were hundreds of Japanese standing in little groups. Many raised clenched fists. Others ostentatiously turned their backs. The sullen resentment of the rest could be inferred. There were disquieting stories of fanatical Japanese continuing to fight after the official surrender. On the other side of the harbour the only building left with two storeys still flew the Japanese flag. It was left alone. Intelligence had advised that up in the hills, well hidden, were twelve Japanese naval guns trained on the harbour. The two goods sheds opposite the wharf were put out of bounds. On our ship in Hong Kong, a few days before, two marines had died after entering a similar building, which had then gone skyward in one searing blast of white flame. There was no leave. Guards were placed on all ships and naval ratings patrolled the wharf. The flagship (a great comfort, a British Cruiser) had preceded us, and the Admiral, with a strong detachment from his staff, had gone inland to the camp.

The whole adventure depended for its success on the final act on the hospital ship and the staff knew this. It was almost all they did know, except that they were to admit an unknown number of patients dangerously ill from undiagnosed diseases and that treatment had to be appropriate and urgent. Gone were the orderly embarkations of Tewfik and Bari with the ambulance convoys, the exact lists, and the detailed case notes. The planning fell into two departments, the administrative under Major Stevely and the clinical under Major Ludbrooke. (Just before Hong Kong, Major O'Regan had been transferred to India and Captain Aitken of Wanganui had replaced him.) The vestibule was transformed into an admitting office. The best wards were made available by moving some of the Hong Kong patients.

Meanwhile there were two incidents. An American plane full of ex-prisoners took off from Tokyo for Manila but failed to evade the cyclone, and eventually came down near a destroyer. The passengers, using parachutes, were strewn over two miles of rough sea. The destroyer did what it could and eventually collected nine survivors of the original twenty-two. Some of them were in bad shape. The destroyer had no medical officer and no facilities and no heart for mercy missions. It made for the nearest port (Keelung) hoping for a ship perhaps with a medical officer. Instead it found the miracle of a hospital ship. It did not negotiate. It dumped its patients on the wharf and made off. So the small group from Japan was embarked and was allotted beds. They were specialists in the art of survival. Daily in their ward they stole sugar from the locked cupboards but always gave it back to Sister, saying it was a harmless instinct they could not resist.

The other incident concerned the Japanese harbour master who came on board and requested audience with the O.C. Troops. He was a squat individual, speaking stilted English, and with a face as bland as the lid of a tin. He expressed his pleasure at the termination of the dreadful war and the coming of the day of universal friendship. He was grieved to hear that some of the poor prisoners had fallen ill. He had brought them some presents. Here he opened a paper bag with matchstick toys, straw rickshaws, paper fans, cardboard wallets. He hoped the presents would take their minds off their illness. For a little his hypocrisy left me speechless. The long chain of islands up the Pacific from Guadalcanal to Keelung all recorded an unvarying tale of Japanese atrocities. We were here to rescue the survivors of an extermination camp. Not all the gewgaws in the world would stifle the memory of mass murder. *Timeo Danaos et dona ferentis.*

I said I would be no party to his attempt to buy an indemnity by such methods. I ordered him off the ship and to take his trash with him and never come back. He went, unabashed and unemotional, bearing himself with the irritating impassivity of an Oriental.

The next day the Admiral came back. There were nearly two hundred patients. They were seriously ill. Diagnosis? Starvation – so they all said. 'Though they don't look starved to me.' There was a dreadful apathy about some. One man had died while he was there. But the majority were absorbed with the drama of their rescue. Never in their dreams had they imagined a hospital ship round that desolate coast. And why of all places in the world should it have come from New Zealand?

'They asked me,' said the Admiral, 'whether you had nurses on board. I said the New Zealand Government had combed the country for the best and prettiest nurses they could find – all for them. You have nurses, I hope?'

'Yes. They may not be exactly as you describe but you're remarkably close.'

At last, on time, the train appeared through a cleft in the hills. It was driven by two naval ratings who had once had a vague connection with railways. The two Japanese drivers had not been co-operative and had been beaten up and thrown off.

The rain had ceased and the cyclone had thinned to a bitter wind. Slowly the black chain of boxlike little carriages drew up into the ruins of Keelung, then reversed and came down the wharf and stopped opposite the ship. The marines came forward with stretchers. The first patients were carried up. They were hidden under blankets, face and all, for the cold journey across the wharf. In the vestibule there was a rapid examination. After the first dozen or two the main pattern became clear.

The most striking feature was the famine oedema such as no one on that ship had ever seen before. They were bloated all over. Malnutrition spares no organs. There were grossly defective livers and kidneys, anaemia without exception and every known avitaminosis except scurvy. The most urgent need was a drip infusion of plasma to build up the blood proteins. That, and food, and nursing, and faith again in the dignity of human existence. Inevitably there would be chronic infections, malaria, hookworm, tuberculosis, diabetes – all these could wait.

In the vestibule Major Ludbrooke and his staff worked at high pressure. The ward allocation had to respect ease of exit in emergencies, ward facilities for treatment, stability in rough seas. Mistakes could become disasters.

As the routine became established each stretcher took less than a minute to go through the formula of admission in the crowded vestibule. Our orderlies took the stretchers to the allotted ward with the indications for treatment already outlined. The last stretchers went up in the late afternoon. The train chugged up to the head of the harbour and was there abandoned. The Japs who had moved down the hill behind its screen now moved back. The early part of the embarkation had been witnessed by the Admiral. When it was well over he came back.

'Well,' he said, 'How are you getting on?'

I invited him to see. The vestibule was almost clear again. We went down the broad companion-way to Ward D. Halfway down he stopped with an exclamation of astonishment.

It was indeed a sight to halt the step, to stay the voice. The ward, once the main lounge, spread the width of the ship. It was low-decked, painted cream and was ablaze with a mass of lights. All the cots, many of them swinging on chains, were occupied. The patients had been bathed or sponged, had been stripped of the last of their rags and were in new pyjamas. They lay under coloured counterpanes between white sheets on soft mattresses. Many had an arm exposed and into the vein plasma was running. The full staff was there – medical officers, Sisters, VADs, ward sergeants, orderlies – but they moved without fuss or haste. The only sound was a low murmur compounded of many quiet activities with no voice above a conversational level.

They were finishing their meal. Each patient had his tray. They had small appetites as yet but they could marvel at the choice. Fish, lamb, poultry, root vegetables, potatoes, custard, fruit, milk, cream, cheese, sugar, salt – how good in the world of created things is honest food.

The Admiral moved round among them. The day before, he had seen them lying on bamboo poles with no mattress and covered with one blanket. Now they had little to say, lacking appropriate words. A few gave him a commendatory nod, as if to say that though they hadn't believed him he had been right after all. One or two held up white bread and butter as if only high rank could confirm the miracle. A few were asleep. One or two were dying.

But the emotionalism of the men had roots beyond the material matters of facilities and amenities. It was based on the presence of the Matron and her band of quiet, efficient Sisters and VADs, thereby complementing the deep spiritual needs of segregated men. In all their dreams in captivity, women had figured in the abstract as a corollary to their rehabilitation. But now everything had been reversed. The abstract had yielded to an astonishing reality. The women had come almost to the threshold of the copper mines to initiate the rehabilitation rather than add a postscript to it. In their traditional role of healing where men had caused the bruising they brought all the resources of nursing and laughter, soothing and chiding and dextrous hands. All these – but the greatest of all was compassion.

'We'll get out of this hell-hole tomorrow,' said the Admiral.

But on the morrow the seas were still rough and some men were close to death. I intervened. The Admiral agreed. The *Maunganui* stayed, with one destroyer. The others left, the last signal from the flagship expressing farewell and appreciation. Their departure made the place even more eerie. As dusk fell there were still groups of Japs half a mile away on the hills. Perhaps we would have been safer far out to sea. That evening, out of the silence so deep it could have been ominous, a rifle was fired near the foot of the gangway. Almost immediately there was a second shot. Members of the staff and crew raced to the gangway. We were met not by Japanese aggression but by British embarrassment. The guard on the gangway admitted to a nervous dislike of the whole environment. In this mood his rifle had accidently discharged. His mate, a few yards away, had been unable to inhibit the reflex and had also fired. We left them to an irate naval officer. At least the Japs now knew that we were armed and alert.

The next morning, no considerations of weather would keep us any longer in Formosa. As we moved out, with Captain Prosser manoeuvring the ship round the small harbour as if it were a badly parked car, the Japs came running down to the wharf. Their farewell was as stereotyped as their welcome had been. Some shook their fists. Others turned their backs bent forward and dropped their pants. This was meant to be a humiliating insult of withering intensity. On the *Maunganui* it produced the same effect as a vaudeville act, spoilt only by the target being out of range of a boot. Outside the harbour we swung from the coast into the deep, clear, plunging, green seas.

Yet – for me anyhow – the triumph was blurred. The next day a paper bag addressed to me was found in a remote corner of the deck. It contained the toys donated by the Keelung harbour master to the dear patients. I conducted a savage enquiry which proved that the toys had gone off the ship with him but which failed to reveal how they had got back. Ruefully I had to admit that after two rounds he was leading on points. In the end I told the story in *Whatknots* and set the display out on the deck. It was then at the mercy of anyone. Slowly it began to disappear and then quite rapidly it was gone – overboard most likely.

Early one morning there was tramping and shuffling on the deckhead above my cabin. All the patients from Formosa and Japan who could limp had assembled there. Led by their indomitable Padre Pugh they were participating in a commemorative service, for here, close to Manila, was where the Americans had bombed the Japanese convoy, half of which contained prisoners battened down. This the Americans knew but the Japs had changed the signs and the wrong ships were bombed. Those at the commemoration were some survivors.

We came to Manila, primarily for oil. There was oil there, but not enough for the vast concourse of moving vessels. Our claim was only the mute appeal of our red crosses. Wellington had lost us, America had never heard of us; the British Navy had granted us independence and sent us off. Captain Prosser began sleuthing tankers. He weaved a course through Manila harbour, reminiscent of the flight of a hesitant moth. The tanker he was pursuing came alongside a British destroyer and with nautical expertise the *Maunganui* swept up on the other side and stayed. Our tanks began to fill. The officers of the destroyer invited any of our ambulant naval officers to lunch. Shortly after, I was informed that the R.N. refused to go if the R.N.V.R. went also. Would I rule? I was first astonished, and then angry. In Fairview a spade was a spade and in Blackball a shovel was a shovel and in the Pacific a bit of damn nonsense was a bit of damn nonsense. I ruled. Either they all went or none went and they had five minutes to decide. They all went.

Meanwhile we had contacted the *Oxfordshire*, laden with the rest of the Hong Kong patients. It was bound for England. We were bound for New Zealand. The patients were not consulted as to their destination. It happened then that wives might be on one ship and husbands on another. It was too late to change, said the navy, forgetting that it had given us in effect an independence which we had no intention of wasting. The two O.C.s Troops conferred. I sent an officer to the *Oxfordshire* with a boat load of sight-seeing patients. He returned with an equal number but they were not the same persons. We embarked a few more patients at Manila. Only then did we begin to prepare the master rolls of those on board.

Sydney was over three thousand nautical miles away and it was going to be too long a voyage for some. The bloated bodies would remain bloated until relieved by a massive urinary flow which would not start till a certain level of protein in the blood had been reached. Our initial standard treatment then was to boost these proteins by intravenous plasma. Most fortunately we had on this voyage Captain Doyle, a stalwart pathologist from Auckland. He guided us by doing hundreds of serum protein estimations. The practice became so routine that every orderly would glance at the report and say to the patient, 'You're coming on nicely, old man. Another couple of days and you'll start'. In addition to our large supplies of plasma, Major Ludbrooke had some precious blood flown in from Okinawa by the Americans. Unpredictable people, the Americans. At Manus, where we stopped briefly, two American officers offered me an enormous amount of plasma, so cheap that I was immediately suspicious and insisted on seeing it. Reluctantly they showed me. The plasma was in the jungle in a pile of rotting cartons. Many bottles were smashed and in some of the others lumpy precipitates moved in a milky medium. I suspect the officers were quartermasters in trouble with their accounting.

No one on the staff had leisure. Hours of duty were nominal only. The medical staff was increased by bringing Captains Blair and Lewis into the officers' mess and allotting them wards. I also took over one ward.

Much of the success of that voyage was due to *Whatknots*. In the vestibule was a postbox in which manuscripts were dropped. This kept me busy for most evenings. The late prisoners were encouraged to write their experiences and some dramatic (and possibly unique) material was produced. One issue reached forty single-spaced foolscap pages. It was a valuable therapeutic agent. The writers, having told the world, felt better. But after three such issues I peremptorily stopped the horror stories. Creeping in were some morbid notes of self-pity. It was the psychological moment to turn full-face to the future.

The two camps from Hong Kong provided an interesting study.

223

Shamsuipo was the military camp where every inmate was a potential escapee, and consequently the control was harsh. But their discipline never faltered. They all shared equally and uncomplainingly. But there was less composure in Stanley Camp where were civilians. They lacked from the start any organization from which discipline would be acceptable. The struggle for survival was therefore a struggle among themselves. Some of these people we could never cure of the habit of hoarding. They would eat to repletion and then slip a couple of pieces of buttered bread into a handkerchief or a handbag and then leave them to mildew in lockers or drawers.

On a bright sunny afternoon the ship, striking in its white and red against the olive-green hills and the battle-grey of ocean liners, sailed up the Sydney harbour. At one point it seemed to catch up with a celebration on shore. Flags were being run up, sirens, whistles, hooters were sounding. It was taken up on the opposite side of the harbour. We were only mildly curious. Australians often had quixotic interests. Perhaps the Melbourne Cup . . . . Then we found that the clamour along the harbour's shores moved as we moved, and in a sudden moment of revelation we knew that this was Sydney's welcome to our patients. And – on thinking it over – why not? The ultimate, in war, aims to rescue the prisoners from the arrogant enemy. Operation Pacific had been completed by the British, American, New Zealand and Australian services with the supporting bases in Australia. Over the water came fresh bursts of cheering.

We passed under the bridge. Everybody knew of course of the extraordinary optical illusion whereby for a few seconds the bridge is going to snap off the ship's mast or the mast is going to cleave the bridge. It was anticipated with much jocularity but as the bow went under the bridge a sudden silence fell. A voice said anxiously, 'Ba goom, ther cap'in's been and gone and done it naow'. At the time, I was standing at the foot of the mast. When we passed I was almost the only one there. All the others had instinctively moved to the scuppers.

We were at Sydney only long enough to leave a few patients and embark a lesser number. In the Tasman there was the usual grand occupational therapy exhibition, with Miss Cullen arranging her arrogant Donald Ducks and submissive koala bears. *Whatknots* produced its final copy and officially farewelled the patients. A few more came up from the wards to join the growing number of ambulants.

In these last few days the voyage could be assessed. All the voyages had been successful but this one was the greatest triumph because of the greater obstacles. The real drama had been in the wards where death was never far from any cot. Seven died on the voyage, which meant that out of every hundred, there were ninety-eight survivors, a record of which we could be proud. In each instance death, within the scope of our facilities, was inevitable.

The credit belonged to the whole ship. There was total loyalty to a cause which meant loyalty to each other. The orderlies and N.C.O.s set a standard. They worked uncomplainingly for long hours, slept in crowded and often stifling conditions, had no place of retreat and a minimum of amenities. The Sisters, of course, were splendid. In my ward one evening I handed Sister a list of the patients due for intravenous transfusion in the morning. And she asked, if you're late, shall I start? But despite her expertise and her love of exploiting it, the drips were my responsibility. I would not be late, I said. But, she persisted, you just might; anyone working as hard as you . . . . This was a piece of blarney for which she should have been smacked. Instead, I agreed that if I was not there by 0930 hours she could start. The next morning I aimed at punctuality but something befell and I arrived ten minutes late. All fourteen drips were running smoothly. Quite obviously she had not done them all in ten minutes, but when I enquired among the patients and staff, half of them seemed to have forgotten to wind their watches and the other half had a patchy amnesia. This is a loyalty which transcends veracity. Secretly I approved of it.

But perhaps the major credit for the success of that voyage goes to the patients. Even a few given to carping would have destroyed the harmony. Perhaps the affinity between them and the staff would not have been possible if they had come to us under less emotional circumstances. But, as it was, it was a rich experience for all involved. I have still a file of appreciative letters all spontaneously delivered. One, from Ward H, is signed by every patient. They are too numerous and too lengthy to quote but an arresting feature is the frequent reference to New Zealand. 'This has been our first experience of New Zealanders and, sir, if you will allow me to use a Scots expression they are "grand people". I don't think one of us on this ship will ever forget the kindness we have received from all.' 'When I left my own ship it was my last thought that I should be going to a N.Z. ship. All doubts about finding it strange were dispelled in the first 24 hours and I found instead a friendliness that was hard to imagine.' '. . . Our deep appreciation and grateful thanks for the many kindnesses and courtesies of the sisters and nurses of the N.Z. Nusing Services and the officers and other ranks of the N.Z.M.C.' '. . . And to sense again the natural courtesy, kindliness and friendship that is to be found in the outside world and nowhere more readily than in our own N.Z. corner of it.'

There was also a collective effort. From their meagre resources the patients arranged for the supply of a plaque at Wellington.

> Presented by the liberated prisoners of war and internees from Hong Kong, Japan and Formosa in gratitude for the sympathetic and generous treatment which they received from the hospital staff and ship's complement on H.M.N.Z.H.S. *Maunganui*.
> Sept. – Oct. 1945.
> 'I was sick, and ye visited me: I was in prison, and ye came unto me.' – Matthew 25:36.

In Wellington it was fitting that the British High Commissioner, Sir Patrick Duff, should board the ship out in the harbour and that the Governor-General, Sir Cyril Newall, should be waiting on the wharf. In the Casualty Clearing Station the patients were welcomed on behalf of the Government and the people. Even we, authorities on administrative technique, had no fault to find with the arrangements at Wellington. The cot cases, the metabolic tragedies, went by hospital train, some to Palmerston North but mostly to the Hutt Hospital. For the majority it was their last journey for, after two years, there were few survivors.

The ambulant ones were for a few hours given the freedom of the city of Wellington, and in the New Zealand tradition already started, lacked nothing. But that evening they were back on the ship and the next morning were in the Convalescent Depot at Burnham (where, as a delicacy, they were given rice). Thereafter Burnham was a postal address only. All leave was granted as applied for. They had very little money but they seemed to need even less. They roamed the country from Auckland to Invercargill. They were grand ambassadors for the country of their hosts. Then, after a month, the majority were back on the *Maunganui* again and the wards were filled with other refugees from Hong Kong brought to Auckland by the *Tjitzalengka*.

The last voyage of the *Maunganui* was to England and back. But all the glory had gone. Many patients were exchanged at Melbourne for less able ones. Strangers predominated. Our staff had changed. Major Stevely, Major Ludbrooke, R.Q.M. Scully and some of the senior Sisters and veteran O/Rs had gone. Their substitutes knew nothing of hospital ships, nor recognized any incentive to learn. There were new faces at ports of call. Only at Perth was the Red Cross as magnificent as ever.

After Christmas on board, a deputation of Scottish officers, late prisoners in Formosa, informed me that Hogmanay was due in a few days. This was the first time for years that they might be able to celebrate it as it should be celebrated. Would I give permission for a midnight party? I considered their last Hogmanay. Every man who had not filled his quota of copper ore was stripped to his loin cloth, made to clasp a pole above his head and was thrashed on the back by a pumpkin-faced Jap. Certainly they could have their midnight party. They warned me that this would involve whisky in bottles which was outside the rules. Not if they negotiated with the chief steward and I heard no whisper of it. Thank you sir, and as it was an exclusive party could they borrow my cabin – in fact both rooms, bedroom and office? Yes certainly (I could probably go and read in the orderly room). Thank you again, sir, and now would you honour us by being our guest. Here I began to feel for the brake. If I went on like this they would soon be serving me up like an Aztec sacrifice. I said I had never been in Scotland in my life, that I did not like whisky, that I had no idea what was the derivation of Hogmanay (nor had they, I discovered later) and that, despite my rank, I was only a faceless Sassenach. Not so, they all assured me. Their arguments were multiple and persuasive even though not very logical. In the end, overwhelmed but unconvinced, I agreed.

I left the cabin in the late evening and went back half an hour before midnight. I could hardly get in. The place was full of braw bodies talking, drinking, with some wearing artificial thistles and others with fragments of tartan. I was noisily welcomed and had a glass pressed on me. It was full of pale amber liquid. In the tradition of Hogmanay they assured me I had to drink it straight off. I had no intention of drinking it straight off. I had been on too many ships where the planned procedure of the mess was to drink a newcomer under the table. I suspected a whisky-drenched ambush. But it was not whisky. On the contrary it was rather pleasant. And they were all good chaps. They were pained at my suspicion. Only at Glencoe have guests of the Scots been in danger. So I drank it off. As I put the glass down they were all watching and there seemed a sudden relaxation, almost a sigh of relief. For about ten minutes there ensued the social obligations of talk. Then I found myself agreeing with the last speaker, and the next, and embracing everyone's point of view. Some of the men about me began to sway and the table swayed with them. Yet through the open door the sea was calm. Was anything wrong with the ship, I asked aloud. A chorus assured me that everything was all right. I was not quite so sure. I knew more of the sea than they did. Anything can happen at sea.

But they were magnificent hosts. Always at my hand was a full glass and if I took a social sip now and then it was replenished before I could remove my hand. At midnight a tall, dark and mysterious figure entered slowly through the cabin door. Everyone applauded, including myself. It seemed the right thing to do as it seemed the right thing to laugh when they all laughed. Later, during a less somnolent phase, I proposed a toast to

'Bonnie Scotland' which was enthusiastically received. Then they began drifting off. First-footing, so I understood. I went second-footing to bed. In the morning the cabin was clean, brushed and swept. Some of them told me it was the greatest Hogmanay party they had ever known. Good. In such circumstances there was a little satisfaction in being the licensing authority, despite the headache.

It was a weary and harassing voyage of what had once been a hospital ship and was now a liner. We arrived at long last at a pier at Southampton where everyone ignored us. I went ashore. Yes, they knew we were there; they were trying to arrange accommodation for our patients. Disembarkation would probably start early in the evening. And then could I give leave to my staff? Certainly not. No leave in Southampton. The trains to London were being maintained with great difficulty. They gave me books of blank leave passes but only after I promised not to use any in the vicinity of Southampton.

They left us late that night, the last of our old patients from the Pacific, a slowly moving file down the gangway to a troop train that would take them off to some inland camp. There was no flag flying, no band, no cheers, no relatives nor friends. Truly the British are a strange people. Because of their fortitude and endurance these men had brought glory to the British name on the far side of the earth and Britain had welcomed them back with petulance at their inopportune arrival. Perhaps the relatives were not informed, perhaps they were not allowed to travel. But surely at least one flag might have been flown, one speech might have been made to the survivors of the copper mines. This place, to my mother, was home. I thought of the welcomes at Sydney and Wellington. It was not home to me.

We sailed that night, a disgruntled staff in an empty, untidy cheerless ship. The next morning we dropped anchor at the mouth of the Thames. The cold was of the penetrating type that New Zealand never knows. Again we were ignored. We were waiting for orders, said Captain Prosser. And if they did not come? Then we stayed at the mouth of the Thames. For the first time on the ship I had to placate a difficult staff, or rather those few members who, now the war was over, were overseas for the first time. From an office on a pier at Southend, I rang Brigadier Twhigg, last seen in New Caledonia and now working with Brigadier Kippenberger and Colonel Rudd in the repatriation of prisoners. I said I could hear, far-off, the rumblings of a meeting. He promised to do what he could. Back on the ship, I sensed trouble. So I called the whole staff together, told all I knew and asked for their co-operation and sense of fairness. It was a good speech and would probably have been successful had it not been interrupted in midflight by a message from the Master. A pilot was on his way to take us up the Thames.

Later in the day we were up in the docks, anchored in mid-stream. At length the customs came aboard and went through our declarations. Everyone had too many cigarettes. What would we prefer? Pay duty or leave them on the ship? Leave them on the ship, elected everyone. Then customs disappeared into the shadows presumably to lie in wait till the shore authorities would permit our disembarkation. The cold, if possible, bit deeper. On the other side of the ship a barge drifted up. Some of our more experienced N.C.O.s opened negotiations out of earshot. A rope was thrown, the barge came alongside. Men piled on to its deck and helped the nursing staff aboard. The rest followed, baggage, cigarettes and all. The barge churned off and landed us at a deserted wharf on the other side of the dock. He was a good man, that bargeman, the sort of man who almost certainly would have been at Dunkirk. He received some compensation underwritten by regimental funds. There was a rush through the dock gates which brought the gate-keeper, his mouth full of a meal, limping out of his lodge and protesting that the charge was a shilling a head. He looked disconsolately after the invading force which by now was well out in the freedom of London. So I gave him a pound and he went back to his meal.

After a few days private visiting in Devon and Winchester, I came back to London. Most of the days were spent with Brigadier Twhigg trying to anticipate the problems of the return voyage. Problems indeed. Half the ship was to be for hospital cases and half for passengers. We were to take many wives of New Zealand soldiers and a number of babies. For the babies, our only accommodation was a jumble of cots and a playroom. For their mothers we could offer only dormitory accommodation with a communal wardrobe and little else. I drafted a letter which went to all women on our list. It depreciated the ship as a passenger ship, detailed its defects and suggested they withdrew unless they were prepared to accept austere conditions without complaint. About a dozen withdrew and their places were immediately taken.

Eventually we sailed, as full and as varied as Noah's Ark and, like it, hoping to endure the waters for the next forty days and nights. But we had greater problems than those of Noah. The first item of a mass of official mail awaiting me was from the Admiralty. It stated that recently too many mental patients on hospital ships had been lost overboard. This must stop. . . . We had a locked ward for about twelve. Actually we had thirty-two known psychiatric cases. In the ward we kept the most suicidal, changing them according to their swings of mood. We lost none, good fortune prevailing where good organization was impossible. One patient had a favourite spot outside my cabin. He would rehearse the preliminary stages of going overboard, knowing I was watching. This was bluff, but bluff is often a treacherous mask. He was, however, shadowed by a friend explaining the risk and the precautions to take. I discovered a few days later that the patient was at large and the friend was in the psychiatric ward. On another occasion I unlocked the door of this ward. A burly patient rushed at me, bounced off and began to clamber over the rail. I collared him in a rugby tackle and held him long enough for the sergeant to arrive.

At first the voyage followed predictable lines. The Bay of Biscay was rough and the new passengers surrendered more or less *en masse*. In the Mediterranean the first sun showed. We sailed between Italy and Sicily (Scylla and Charybdis). This was exciting. I was invited to the bridge and there, with binoculars, could see into the Sicilian houses perched on the cliffs. At Bari we embarked more patients. We also embarked Lieutenant-Colonel C. Burns again who was to be our senior physician. He was to me a great support. He soon had all the difficult medical cases under control and then, as is his wont, began to organize clinical meetings for medical officers. There was the excitement of the canal and the ports at either end. By then we had our full quota of army (one hundred and fifty-three), navy (fourteen), airforce (fourteen), wives (one hundred and twenty-three), Waacs (five), civilians (forty-seven), babies (twenty-four), children (one). It could have been a prickly group even apart from the terrific heat of the Red Sea. Exhausted mothers could not deal with their babies and had to hand them over to the nursing staff. All the babies had heat rashes. Our fans were ineffective and there was no air conditioning. Furthermore, about seventy of our women patients were pregnant, some in the last trimester.

The passengers adjusted to the difficult conditions by the traditional method of finding a scapegoat. The scapegoat in this instance was an amorphous authority vaguely referred to as 'They'. They had cramped them, ill-fed them, underventilated them. The list went on enlarging. The local representatives of 'They' were the Master and myself and our respective officers.

Captain Prosser stated with conviction that all passengers who embarked on a ship went mad. (He sometimes added that they had been mad before that, otherwise they would never have gone on a ship.) Some women (a few only) became rude and abusive. Nominally it was still an army unit. I could discipline the men and on that voyage held several orderly rooms. But I had no authority over the women – unless any of them came into labour in which case I suppose I, as senior obstetrician, would have had to change battledress for gown and exercise authority of a different sort.

Yet, after all, it mattered little. Most of the staff were good-humoured and efficient. At Tewfik I needed a new Adjutant and appointed one of the patients, Lieutenant-Colonel D. G. Kennedy, afterwards Director-General of Health. He filled the position admirably. The ship became taut with discipline. If I met him suddenly I had to restrain an impulse to salute. The great majority of the patients and passengers were appreciative and said so. (One of the women was discovered, halfway through the voyage, to be a registered medical practitioner.) The babies, all nappied up in their bikinis and rolling over each other on blankets, were delightful. In both wars I had returned to New Zealand on duty among wives and babies. Routine orders came out every day, plasters were changed, the stumps of the amputees were shaped, *Whatknots* appeared regularly, occupational therapy culminated in the usual exhibition at the end of the voyage (The A. & P. Show) and every day brought Wellington nearer.

We were due at Fremantle on a Sunday. I sent a message to the Red Cross asking if they could arrange a picnic. This they did magnificently. Cars and buses were on the wharf and those who filled them had a grand day in the country and came back staggering under a load of fruit. But a number preferred to go into Perth. I had addressed all going ashore on the subject of drink but it was only a request for moderation. I had no heart for an impassioned appeal. Behaviour in the main was good. A few – the same troublesome few – came back noisy and aggressive. When we were ready to sail six persons were missing. We waited and after a while they appeared, three men and three women, all very drunk, reeling along the wharf.

Ten days later we came to Wellington. Dear, lovely Wellington. Disembarkation was the usual orderly confusion. I saw some of the more difficult women fall into the arms of their husbands. I forgave them everything. They too had been under strain. They were leaving 'home' to cast their lot with a man they hardly knew and whose beret they were inclined to mistake for a halo. One is reminded of the English bride of the first war trying to locate a husband who owned a treacle mine in Moray Place, Dunedin, or of the Kiwi of the second war who sold a Cairo tram to an Arab. A Minister of the Crown welcomed them, said he was sure they were glad the voyage was over and hoped that they would never regret becoming New Zealand citizens. Few listened to him. Fewer listened to me in reply.

I had a few days at home and then for a week was back on the ship, now at Evans Bay. Masses of equipment were torn out and I signed innumerable forms. It was a dull and tiring labour, a treadmill sort of activity. But in the evenings, in the vast silence of a near-empty ship, I kept thinking of its enormous past, of its efficiency, humanity, loyalty, ideals and international regard. Yet no one seemed to know of this. The ship had truly become part of the forgotten fleet. It was then I resolved that some record would have to be made – not of a ship merely moving from port to port as Dr T. Duncan Stout has done briefly in his official history of the medical services in the Pacific, but of a ship with a soul, a grand purveyor of the humanities. And this I have attempted in this chapter, poorly, perhaps, but proudly.

One evening a taxi took me to the ferry. I did not see the *Maunganui* again. It took the New Zealand Contingent to the victory march in London. After that, it was sold somewhere in South America. At subsequent ship reunions its further fate is obscured by conflicting rumours. Now even the rumours have stopped.

In *An Encyclopaedia of New Zealand, Vol. III* (Wellington, Government Printer, 1966) there is a section on this country's famous ships. Apparently fame rests on seaworthiness or naval prowess and not on the drama by which New Zealanders came to New Zealand. So there is no mention of the *Bengal Merchant*, the *Phillip Laing*, the *Charlotte Jane* or the *Maunganui*.

11

Après la Guerre

Repatriation in a soldier's career is a splendid bloom erupting from the bud of demobilization, grand for the short space and then dropping its petals, done, gone, finished. It involved the tremulous moment of reunion with fiancée, wife, or parents, a boisterous session with kids, the free railway ticket on which was based the grand tour of aunts and uncles, nephews and nieces. 'We're proud of you boy. You certainly gave them hell. I remember on the Somme. . . .' Back home, the pleasantries piled up, the fervent handshake from the grocer at the corner ('And what are you going to do now?'), a drink with the neighbours across the road, polite cordiality from the strangers on either side. And soon the highlight of repatriation was lost in the long grind of rehabilitation.

The battledress has to go. In the old suit or the patched denims, he wears the camouflage of the civilian. His dependants, if any, now look to him for their needs. He faces a world of competition. The Rehabilitation Department may help him but only he can answer the question, 'What are you going to do now?'

Now, thirty years later, many old soldiers are directed to me by the War Pensions Board. What have they been doing since? A few have built security round their lives. But most, trading work for wage in some small communal niche, have grown older, feebler, in a contracting personal field. Only the family, the R.S.A. and the Pensions Board remember. I search the personal file. They have come from the desert and the jungle, the air and the olive trees, the hills of Greece and Crete. Ichabod, Ichabod. Their rehabilitation was a drift of days with little substance. There is no currency and there never will be any currency that can do justice to the sacrifices of war.

As for me I surveyed without enthusiasm the medical field of Christchurch. There was a host of new doctors, young, energetic, just demobilized, full of ambition and family responsibility. They were where I had been twenty years before. There were old friends, but they were all in a hurry. I visited some nursing homes where there was usually someone who remembered me or pretended to.

What was I going to do now? What I was going to do had been decided long ago in the Pacific. I had been offered a rehabilitation grant. I would go to London, the great medical Mecca and in due time come back to Christchurch, a specialist general physician. More was required than London training but the details have no place here. A housekeeper and her husband moved in. The children promised to be good and off we went, my wife and I, to the lure of London.

Disillusionment began at the wharf in Wellington. I was one in a four-berth cabin, my wife was in a six-berth cabin. I read medicine steadily; my wife knitted and worried over the children at each bedtime. We came to London to a two-roomed flat in the house of friends in North Finchley.

To me, now a sorry civilian, London was a totally different city. There were no staff cars, merely the crush of buses and tubes. We had ration cards which, when mixed with commonsense and economy, prevented hunger without stimulating appetite. The butchers' shops could easily have been adapted to a vegetarian régime.

Weather-wise the year was disastrous. That winter of 1946–1947 established records for cold, snow and ice. It also established records for lack of coal, power, fuel and light.

Of all cities, London must lead in dignity and grandeur. It has a majesty that only a monarchy can give, and a loneliness that only a stranger can know. It is, at times, a city of aesthetic splendour. There have been three times in my life when I have been halted by the sheer beauty of a scene. One was when the sun broke through the London fog and blazoned the Houses of Parliament with chrome and sparkle. Another was in the Inland Philippine Sea where among the spires of the pink and purple mountains a volcano smoked and the shores above the cerulean sea were white with shells. And another was near Bourail, where the grass was sapgreen and the little lake in the centre held the flowering water-lilies and mirrored the mighty flowering frangipani tree at its edge.

In the post-graduate medical world I seemed to share London with half the doctors of the Commonwealth. Many of them, like me, were trying to pick up the clinical threads again. Many others, especially from India, had been civilians during the war and now for the first time were allowed to travel. They were predatory and aggressive. At the post-graduate hospitals the various courses for the next week would be pinned up at known times. As the porter moved back there would be a surging crush from India and Ceylon for the purpose of scribbling a name on every form that could be reached. The number of students was limited, but once a name was down a leisurely choice could be made among the courses that clashed in time. And when a certain attendance became impossible the name might remain and the resultant clinic be short of its quota. I was a Canterbury delegate to the annual B.M.A. conference at Tavistock House, where the formalities included a welcome by the President to the representatives from the Commonwealth. Would any such care to reply? From the far corner of the great hall there was a sudden commotion of chairs capsizing and tables shifting. This was an Indian group each striving to be first at the microphone. No one could question their zeal to learn but many, myself included, felt they could have spread their zeal a little more evenly over the Commonwealth. I had no wish to compete with them.

But there was plenty to do. I attended daily the National Hospital for Nervous Diseases in Queen's Square, did two courses at the West End Hospital for Nervous Diseases, studied chests at Brompton, hearts at Whitechapel, psychiatry at the Maudsley and rheumatic diseases at Bath. There were numerous lectures and demonstrations and frequent visits to the Wellcome Museum. Yet the instruction was not well organized. There were too few available patients and too many doctors. The chaos of the war still obtruded. But it was no fault of the teachers. In famous hospitals I listened to leading men in the medical world and invariably they were friendly, patient, and painstaking in explanation.

One October afternoon in a crush near Euston I saw the posters of the latest editions: 'Sentenced to death – Goering, Von Ribbentrop, Streicher and Keitel. . .' But though I stopped at this vivid compression of history no one else seemed to notice. Crowds came and went, taxis and buses tooted and clanged. There were stacks of papers unguarded by the honesty boxes. This was perhaps the final contempt: the indifference of London to the fate of those who had tried to destroy it. And the noisy bustling activities of the London millions went on unchanged, shortly after, when Goering, no longer able to reach for guns or butter, reached for the cyanide and Ribbentrop, who planned the partition of Europe, was hanged by an American corporal, and Streicher on the scaffold cursed the Jews who were going to survive him and then went to join the six million dead.

After some months, London suddenly palled. It was clogged with motion. All of its millions seemed to be poured into its streets for the purpose of endlessly coming and going. I thought of my section at Motunau on the dreamy North Canterbury plain. Green indeed were the distant fields. The crush and the roar and the nostalgia swept us out of London, but once clear of the smoke we travelled north more slowly, lingering (for such was our mood) at the great cathedrals of Ely, Durham, York and St Giles, till we reached our destination at Aberdeen where for a few fruitful weeks we were the guests of an old friend,

Professor R. S. Aitken (now Sir Robert Aitken of Manchester), Professor of Medicine.

Here, in the Royal Infirmary, was a wealth of clinical material and a freedom of access. It was politic to agree that Aberdeen was a beautiful city, even though the judgement was based on angled roofs and black chimney pots rising above the even surface of the snow. They are hardy, the Scots. I can now understand their devotion to Hogmanay. They are always hoping that the next year will be better than the last. I went into the Royal Infirmary one icy morning just as a filter of a wintry sun broke through. Said the man ahead of me to the porter at the gate:

'Morning Donald. Grand weather we're having now.'

'Aye, Angus, it's a warm morn the morn.'

Back to London, where my wife resumed her restricted domesticity and I returned to Queen's Square and the other haunts. But the adventure was over. Though I knew I would never come this way again it was time to go. Hagley Park, and not Hyde Park, was now calling.

Movement. A week in Paris, where five years of French study at Timaru Boys' High School served us somewhat less well than a week sitting on a kitchen table in a Necal farmhouse talking to a couple of giggling mam'selles might have done; a short holiday in Paignton with the late Dr Stuart Hunter and his wife, a visit to friends at Eastbourne.

A final visit to London, a bag-and-baggage visit. There was no gilt left in London. There were only places and people in the laden streets. I knew of course that in the family life of the homes . . . . But my London was of the streets. There was more human fellowship in the youth who, driving his cows down a Canterbury road, gives a cheerful nod to a stranger than in all the polyglot crush in Piccadilly.

We sailed Thames-Wellington-wise, on the *Largs Bay* which effectively carried passengers from A to B. It had few other virtues except possibly its ability to double the normal occupancy of all its cabins. This time I shared a three-berth cabin with five others. Again, there were many wives of soldiers on board and a large number of children well past the infancy stage. Husbandless mothers, distracted with children on a jammed ship, sweating its way through the Red Sea can make little contribution to harmony. Though I was sorry for the Master it had nothing to do with me. My file was closed. The task allotted me in the interests of shipmanship was to conduct an extended quiz session among the children. They were graded according to their destination in the North or South Island and each such group was subdivided into three by age. Kids are wonderful – if their parents will only leave them alone. When one earnest seven-year-old assured me that the date of Christmas Day in New Zealand was June 25th and I ruled against it, the child's mother attacked me on the grounds of accuracy.

Friends and relations on the Wellington wharf in a day rich with the proximity of home. The ferry that night was a luxury liner and in the morning, beyond the clean and washed hills of Lyttelton, were the kindly plains of Canterbury.

They were all on the station in a little family pocket, the children, my father, kin and friends. How mad and meaningless is the magnificence of a reunion. We reached home. Before going inside I went back and shut the gate.

Christchurch was unchanged in its static outlines but the pace had altered. There were more people, moving more leisurely. There were only a few alien figures in khaki. The week-end now started on Friday night. Saturday morning was strange and barren and splendid. There were no ration books. Fruit could be bought by the case. All that was needed to acquire chocolates was money. Butchers' shops were vulgar in their red, raw variety. A new car which I had not ordered was waiting for me. Christchurch was going to be a nice place. Christchurch thereafter was to be my permanent home.

It was an utterly different medical world. The men had changed. There were numerous new practitioners, nearly all Otago graduates and with new ideas about zoning and group practice and medical centres. Therapy had been vastly invigorated with infusions of narcotics and sedatives, antibiotics, hypotensives, anti-epileptics and the miracle of streptomycin for tuberculous meningitis. Public hospitals and ancillary medical services were free. The patients' fees were subsidized and they paid less and attended more often and the community health improved.

It was the period when the practice of medicine took a forward leap. For the previous century there had been steady progress but only in a continuing tradition. After the war, medicine became deep-rooted in a welfare state nourished by the humanities and politically inviolate. It ceased to be a social artifice dependent on the affluent and charitable, and it acquired mammoth status in a receptive world. New questions began to be asked: about the adequacy of hospitals, of one medical school, of the teaching syllabus, of post-graduate education, of special areas, of improved hospital organization and staffing. There were new facilities for neglected cases, including a great increase in the social service.

But of all the changes the greatest seemed to have been in the patient himself. Often in the old days he had a poor image of the doctor and was inclined to be testy and intolerant. He regarded fee and service as disproportionate. He might even deliver himself of the crushing cliché that he did not believe in doctors.

Now, such types are rarely met. Professional occasions have the leaven of cordiality and the plan of action is often determined by mutual discussion. I might reason with my patient but would not dictate.

Why the change? Most likely, items here and items there. The war levelled out the social strata. There was a new fellowship under the press of national defence and Social Welfare. The patient was now better informed not about the individual doctor but about all doctors. In an emergency any doctor would do. I ask sometimes: 'Who took out your appendix, your gall bladder, your prostrate, your cartilage . . .?' 'Don't know. It was done in the Public. They're all good in there, you know.'

The temptation to enlarge on this must be resisted. Despite the trouble spots in the community and in the world, mankind is steadily ironing out the inequalities in human behaviour. It is a side effect of this that the patient of 1950 was often a more pleasant patient than the one of 1930.

I was re-appointed as Assistant Physician on the hospital staff and was given charge of the infectious diseases and thus was able to supervise the first treatments of tuberculous meningitis with streptomycin. Hospital responsibilities followed: undergraduate and post-graduate education, executive positions on the visiting staff, the library, the staff executive and the founding and control of a clinic on alcoholism. But Canterbury demanded loyalty no less than the hospital. In its centennial year, 1950, I was president of the local division of the B.M.A. and at other times was actively associated with marriage guidance, family planning, the National Society on Alcoholism, the Aged Welfare Council, fund-raising for three hospital chapels, and the board of governors of a private school.

It was pleasant to resume medical lectures to nurses. It was far less pleasant to mark their examination papers at either the local level or in the State Final. My mind would drift; I would start again and read doggedly to the end with my concentration drifting. What is the greater crime in an examination paper, omission of facts or their perversion? How could the undeclared objectives in the minds of examiner and examinee be translated into a fair and just mathematical symbol? A curse on exams. Take a thousand years of compressed knowledge and pick five questions. 'Your pick must be my pick,' says the examiner.

Exams are not in my Utopia. Yet a few examinations presented an occasional bonus. The 'inveterate smoker' in the lecture became the 'invertebrate smoker' in the exam; the best way to diagnose tuberculosis was 'to see puss in the sputum pot'; 'if he was vomiting, his bowel should be kept handy on the locker'; 'on entering the isolation room, the nurse should wear at least a mask'.

Specialism is worthy of the dedication of a whole career. I started too

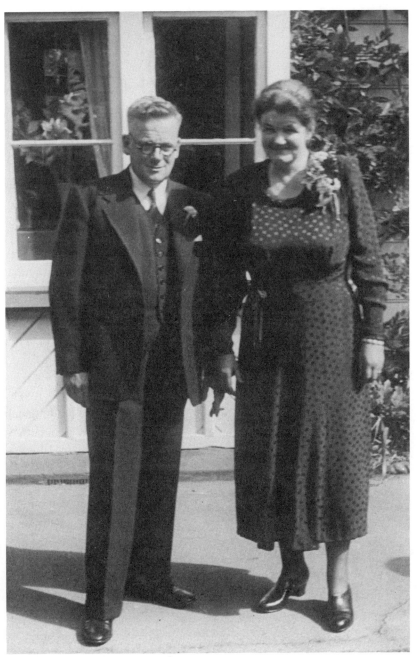

The author and his wife, Christchurch, 1950

late and my subject of general medicine lacked anything comparable to the public image built up around, say, the cardiologist or the neurologist. Yet the aim of specialization is not public esteem; it is to assist the general practitioner. It is an easier life physically, a harder life mentally. The specialist has always to be riding the wave of medical progress.

I had loyal support for many years from small groups of colleagues. Old patients returned. New ventures were made in industrial medicine, pensions, insurances, geriatrics. Constantly, for over forty years, I have been employed by the North Canterbury Hospital Board. Always there has been too much to do.

But here, in 1976, the personal record must end. The thin content of its future will concern mainly health and its deterioration. Ambition, intensity of effort, day-dreaming of achievements – all have gone. It is, in the absence of pain or penury, a mellow time.

Yet the memory of general practice lingers. It forms the very core of the medical world. To the general practitioner is given the title 'my doctor' and to him the summons goes in every crisis. If, in honesty, there is no effective therapy he can declare authoritatively the limit of human resources. He represents the shock troops against disease. There is no substitute for him. While the hazards of human existence persist his need will remain. His day is long, his nights are broken by irruptions into a vast loneliness that has lost the intimacy of the day and replaced it by a distant car-light or the steady futile dance of the traffic signals. He looks for the house with the light and at the bedside has to make a decision on which may depend a life. He works under conditions which no other group in the community would tolerate. It is a jagged existence but usually a limited one. His expectation of life is generally much below that of his patients.

12

The Canterbury Tale

In this, the last chapter, the title needs to be brought forward. For this Canterbury Tale is not my tale. It is a tale of many people, starting with my four grandparents, all scions of the British Isles, who took root in Canterbury and in the tradition of good settlers laboured through long lives in primary and secondary industries, and are now buried in Canterbury soil. Their total of seventeen children is too vast to record. Instead is taken the one example of my own parents. They married and set their feet on the long traditional road of the pioneer. Then came a devastating confrontation with an unrelenting disease. The rest of their story is of the battle they waged, in which they were beaten back . . . and back . . . but because they never lost faith, never despaired and never surrendered, were at the end, battered but triumphant. Out of this struggle I emerged, and my *pot pourri* of detail has to follow chronologically. The story of any locality is the story of the people who lived there. I have avoided autobiography. I have my philosophy, my convictions, my way of life, but I have not the audacity to parade them.

In retrospect, my grandparents' story might be a good story but it can be matched a thousand-fold. Canterbury has been built by its pioneering little family groups, always leaving the cities and the plains better than they found them. My parents, when they retired to upper Armagh Street, had little option. My father could no longer do farm work. He had no pension, no superannuation, no investments. His little surplus cash he used to purchase several decrepit houses where the maintenance (done partly by him but mainly by one of my brothers) was incessant and the rents were precarious. On this, despite his reluctance to accept occasional family assistance, they lived. It was a frugal existence but only in the money sense. Goodwill abounded. All visitors were welcome. It became traditional for them to provide breakfast for all family travellers from the North Island. To my brothers and me it was still home – based on the personality of the two occupants. We did not all share their religious views and the matter was allowed to rest between us. They did not fully understand the work we did, though they were proud of our achievements. (Three of the four sons and seven of the nine grandchildren have university degrees or diplomas.)

Not all valour depends on high adventure. It exists at the domestic levels. The doctors of experience have known of the invalid wife and the husband who attends her, skilfully, cheerfully, persistently. 'I have been glad of the opportunity.' 'It has been a privilege to help her.' 'I think I am fortunate that I am able to do it.' The worth of these men is not in the efforts of today but in their acceptance of tomorrow. They know the incapacity of their partner is permanent and that the road they have taken will not vary in its level monotony. To dedicate themselves to this new life they have to abandon most of the comforting stuff of the old life.

In this select group was my father. His day was as predictable as the seasons – breakfast, housework, my mother's getting-up, reading the paper aloud, gardening, shopping, meals again and the lengthy preparations for bed. Hers was the more protracted day. Even when she was nearly blind she still insisted on doing all the needlework. The radio (a miracle they could never understand) added a little to each day. So did the long telephone conversations with her bed-ridden sister a few streets away. But what each day lacked in activity was filled in each case by the conscious presence of the other.

They had many friends, staunch, steadfast, life-long, of the grappling-with-hoops-of-steel variety, and with a sturdy disrespect of the conventions. The visitors would come in through the open front door, leave the cakes or the scones on the table, shake up the cushions, go and fetch the washing in, make the afternoon tea, bring more cups for late arrivals, and turn the barren afternoon into a joyful occasion. A group of women, amiably disposed, will find an elation in a crossfire of conversation.

My mother never saw a moving picture, and my father only rarely. There was no television. Their travel in the last forty years was to Wellington to my wedding, to Dunedin to the Exhibition, and to Blackball, except for short periods when my mother went to Rotorua. My father attended her daily for over fifty years.

I once realized they had been married for over fifty years. If ever a golden wedding deserved commemoration it was theirs. I went to upbraid them for having forgotten. But they had not forgotten. (My mother, who recorded all the family genealogy in an enormous Bible which I still have, was not likely to have forgotten.) On the appropriate afternoon they had substituted a bottle of port for the teapot and replaced the biscuits with a cream sponge. Here, in an hour or so of reminiscences, they celebrated their golden wedding.

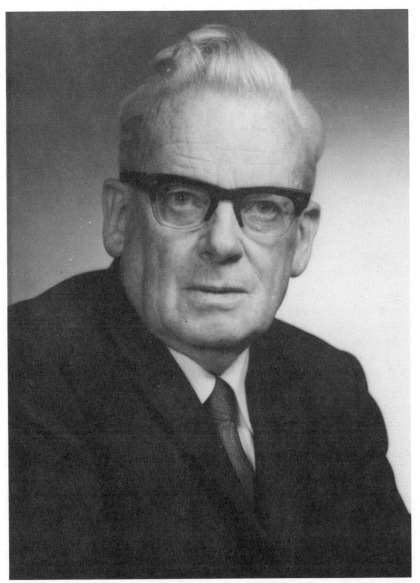

The author, c. 1970

'But, Mother, why on earth. . .?'

'Oh, we weren't going to trouble you. All you boys are so busy. You just leave us alone. We're all right.'

Over the decades their little world contracted, but only at the periphery. The centre was still clean and swept. My father became deafer and stiffer, my mother's sight deteriorated and her frame was grossly distorted. This is the stage when in many families the parents are assumed to have lost all potential and to have transferred all their decisions to their sons and daughters. None of us would have dared. Instead they guided us: a lighthouse, and no flickering candle.

One day, when they were both in their eighties, I was passing the house and a sudden impulse stopped me. As I went up the path I could hear my mother's voice calling in distress. At her feet was lying my father, conscious but unable to get up. Literally, he had worked till he dropped. He was obviously very ill and a short diagnostic term in hospital confirmed that he had not long to live. He came home to the care of professional nurses. When he died my mother, dry-eyed, sat proudly in her chair at the head of his bed. Truly they kept their flag flying.

My mother came to live with me in the special care of my wife. All we could do we did, but we could not replace my father. Again she held her small court. The same friends came and went unannounced. They had the freedom of the bedroom and the bathroom and the kitchen. They were reinforced by the District Nurses and the Foundation for the Blind, generous with their talking books.

Suddenly one day her heart halved its rate. Both I and a medical friend I consulted recognized that in the coming weeks this could be ominous. She, however, forecast her death on the following day and on the following day she died.

I will not write of her death for it was hers and was personal. Our faiths were wide apart at the moment of death, and yet I can think of her death only in her terms: the body raised in incorruption marching in through the open gates and (my addendum) all the bells ringing.

My father, at Fairview, sometimes had to suffer the jibe that he was trying to make his sons better than their father. He certainly tried but he did not succeed.

I once wrote a book on the early colonization of Canterbury, *March of the Little Men* (Wellington, Reed, 1971). That was fiction; the present account is factual. Common to both is the land. Over the face of it the persons come and go and come again, but the land remains, solid and immutable, keeping pace with this moment of eternity. Through my study window the sun is setting and the nor'-west arch is ablaze. The greens, the greys, the purples and the lambent golds lie broadly on estuary and plains, on moutains and sea. Soon will come the new burst of the morning. The last word is always with the land. This has been my place, my home, in whose freedom I have thankfully dwelt a space, filled my days and written my lines.

Chronology

1898	Francis Oswald Bennett born on 19 February in Christchurch
1898–1907	Early childhood spent in Woodbury, South Canterbury
1903	Attended Sydenham School, Christchurch
1906	Attended Woodbury School
1907	Attended Timaru Main School
1907	Moved to Fairview
1907–1911	Attended Fairview School
1912–1916	Attended Timaru Boys' High School
1917	First year student at Medical School, University of Otago
1918	Army, New Zealand and England
1919–1925	Medical training, Medical School, University of Otago
1926–1927	House surgeon, New Plymouth Hospital
1927	Married Pearl Allan Brash
1927–1928	General medical practice in Te Aroha
1928	Birth of first child, Margaret Allan
1928–1933	General medical practice on West Coast
1930	Birth of Jonathan Francis
1932	Birth of Gerald Malcolm
1933	Moved to Christchurch
1933–1940	General medical practice in Christchurch
1937	Birth of Colin Richard
1940–1945	Army, New Zealand, Pacific and Far East
1942	Birth of Kathleen Lorna
1946–1947	Post-graduate study in London
1948–1976	Specialist medical practice in Christchurch
1962	Published *Hospital on the Avon: The History of Christchurch Hospital 1862–1962* (Christchurch, North Canterbury Hospital Board)
1966	Published *The Tenth Home* (Auckland, Blackwood and Janet Paul)
1971	Published *March of the Little Men* (Wellington, A. H. & A. W. Reed)
1976	Wrote *A Canterbury Tale*; died in Christchurch

Glossary

Adrenalin: hormone secreted by the adrenal glands; formerly used in treatment of acute attacks of asthma to open the bronchi

Aneurin: Vitamin B1

Anti-epileptics: drugs used in the control of epilepsy

Aspiration (of pleural effusion): Insertion of needle to draw off pleural fluid

Avitaminosis: lack of a specific vitamin

Bacilliary dysentery: profound diarrhoea, with blood-loss, caused by a bacillus

Bilateral: occurring on both sides

Bromide: a sedative

Cerebro-spinal: affecting brain and spinal cord

Chloral hydrate: a sedative

Chronic: long-lasting

Congestion: accumulation of blood or fluid

Emphysema: chronic lung disorder, characterized by shortness of breath

Erythema nodosum: rare skin disorder, with painful swellings on shins, usually clears up spontaneously within a few weeks

Famine oedema: fluid retention, due to lack of protein

Hypotensives: drugs used in treatment of raised blood pressure

Ileum: part of bowel, at end of small intestine

Intravenous: (of drug) into the vein

Marasmus: wasting away of body

Materia medica: remedial substances used in practice of medicine

Meningism: presence of symptoms of meningeal irritation, i.e. stiff neck, often as symptom of pneumonia

Meningitis: inflammation of meninges, or covering of brain; caused by virus, amoeba or bacteria, latter two forms often fatal

Mitral stenosis: disorder of the heart where the mitral valve (between the left ventricle and left atrium) doesn't open freely. Symptoms of fluid in the lungs and swelling in the periphery

Morbidity: disease

Neuritis: inflammation of the nerves

Osteo-arthritis: degenerative arthritis, usually occurring in the elderly

Peripheral: occurring at the periphery or extremities of the body

Peritoneal cavity: where the gut is situated

Phenobarbitone: a barbiturate used as a sedative

Phthisis: progressive wasting disease, especially pulmonary tuberculosis

Plasma: colourless liquid part of the blood

Pleural effusion: fluid released by lungs through the pleura, or membranes covering the lungs, into the chest cavity (between the lungs and the chest wall)

Popliteal space: area behind the knee

Primapara: woman having her first child (c.f. primagravida – first pregnancy)

Proglottides: propagative segments of tapeworm

Prophylactic: preventive

Puerperal sepsis: infection associated with childbirth, formerly with serious consequences

Pulmonary: of the lungs

Pulp infections: infections of fingers

Quinsies: severe complications of tonsillitis

Rheumatoid arthritis: a severe form of arthritis or inflammation of the joints, with deforming effect, attacks younger people than does osteo-arthritis, characterized by acute phases and periods of remission

Sarcoidosis: disease of unknown cause having its most important effect on the lungs where lumps of tissue (granulomas) form. Formerly thought to be related to TB

Scarlet fever: a streptococcal infection

Scrub typhus: a bacterial infection, similar to typhoid

Sepsis: infection

Septic: infected

Serum protein estimation: an investigation of the blood proteins, to pinpoint cause of oedema

Silicosis: lung fibrosis caused by inhalation of dust containing silica

Slipped ligature: slipped stitch after operation, leading to internal bleeding

Streptococcus: a kind of bacteria

Streptomycin: an antibiotic

Subphrenic: under the diaphragm

Sulphaguanadine: an antibiotic

Suppurative: pus-producing

Tabes (dorsalis): deformity of foot, resulting from tertiary syphilis

Tenosynovitis: inflammation of tendons

Glossary

Tuberculosis: an infection caused by tubercle bacillus, usually in the lungs

Tuberculous meningitis: meningitis caused by tubercle bacillus

Volatile anaesthetics: liquid anaesthetics which readily become gaseous, e.g. chloroform, c.f. gaseous anaesthetics such as nitrous oxide